CARDIOLOGY RESEARCH AND CLINICAL DEVELOPMENTS

HYPERTROPHIC CARDIOMYOPATHY

CAUSES, TREATMENT AND RESEARCH

Cardiology Research and Clinical Developments

Additional books in this series can be found on Nova's website under the Series tab.

Additional e-books in this series can be found on Nova's website under the e-Books tab.

CARDIOLOGY RESEARCH AND CLINICAL DEVELOPMENTS

HYPERTROPHIC CARDIOMYOPATHY

CAUSES, TREATMENT AND RESEARCH

IKRAM KAMMOUN
EDITOR

nova
biomedical
New York

Library of Congress Cataloging-in-Publication Data

ISBN: 978-1-53613-003-4

Published by Nova Science Publishers, Inc. † New York

CONTENTS

INTRODUCTION

Iacopo Olivotto*, MD
Head, Cardiomyopathy Unit
Careggi University Hospital
Florence, Italy

Hypertrophic cardiomyopathy, universally known as HCM, has never ceased to fascinate physicians and scientists since its first modern description in the early 1950s by Donald Teare in London. As a tangible result of such fascination, impressive progress has been achieved and it is undeniable that the outlook of HCM patients and their families today is significantly more favorable than originally perceived. The last 20 years have witnessed a true paradigm shift in HCM perception from the "rare and malignant" condition described in the 1970s and 1980s at several international referral centers, to the "not-so-rare and relatively benign" disease depicted by a wealth of literature based on less-selected patient populations and community hospitals. Most HCM patients today can aspire to normal longevity and a good quality of life.

It is equally undeniable, however, that despite an accelerating accumulation of knowledge on its molecular and clinical profile, HCM is

* Corresponding Author: iacopo.olivotto@gmail.com.

under-diagnosed in the community and remains an orphan disease, lacking specific therapies capable of impacting its natural history. To date, many aspects of this disease remain poorly understood and constitute a 'mystery'. These include the extreme variability in phenotype (even within the same family), the lack of meaningful genotype-phenotype correlations, the triggers of disease progression towards the hypokinetic or restrictive phase and the determinants of arrhythmic propensity, just to name a few. State-of-the-art treatment is based on old pharmacological agents, mainly aimed at controlling symptoms and arrhythmias, use of an implantable defibrillator for primary or secondary arrhythmic prevention and surgical or percutaneous intervention to relieve dynamic outflow obstruction. Transplants are done but rarely needed.

Thus, large gaps in knowledge as well as in awareness remain. On one hand, it is important to spread the idea that HCM is a common disease and a major determinant of cardiovascular morbidity in the young, warranting earlier and broader identification within the community. On the other hand, it is crucial to expand the horizons of HCM research and excellence in clinical management, to include novel institutions and geographical areas and reach a capillary diffusion of cardiomyopathy literacy worldwide.

It therefore gives me great pleasure to introduce "Hypertrophic Cardiomyopathy: Causes, Treatment and Research" edited by Dr. Ikram KAMMOUN, which provides a concise but comprehensive overview of the most important issues pertaining to diagnosis, risk stratification and management of HCM. In an up-to-date overview ranging from diagnosis and genetic testing to invasive management of obstruction, this book offers a wealth of scientific insights and clinical guidance to all those involved in the care of HCM patients.

The community of HCM patients and their families deserve to find excellence at their door-step, and not only at a few international centers. This book is a significant step forward in the right direction.

In: Hypertrophic Cardiomyopathy
Editor: Ikram Kammoun
ISBN: 978-1-53613-003-4

Chapter 1

RECENT ADVANCES IN GENETIC TESTING FOR HYPERTROPHIC CARDIOMYOPATHY

Sinda Zarrouk-Mahjoub[1,*], Josef Finsterer[2], Mouna Hadj Brahim[1] and Ikram Kammoun[3]

[1]Genomics Platform, Pasteur Institute of Tunis, Tunis ElManar University,Tunis, Tunisia
[2]Krankenanstalt Rudolfstiftung, Vienna, Austria
[3]Department of cardiology, Tunis ElManar University, Ariana, Tunisia

ABSTRACT

Hypertrophic cardiomyopathy (HCM) is a primary disease of the myocardium that occurs mainly due to mutations in gene encoding for proteins of the cardiac sarcomere. HCM, the most common familial form of cardiomyopathy, is inherited in an autosomal dominant pattern, and presents with variable expressivity and age-related penetrance. The pathophysiology of HCM is complex, being characterized by a wide range of disease processes, with varying genetics, clinical manifestations, heart morphology and function, response to treatment, prognosis, and outcome. In any case, molecular diagnosis of HCM is of paramount importance, since it may make it possible to detect subjects carrying

* Corresponding Author: sinda.zarrouk@pasteur.tn.

mutations on HCM-associated genes before they develop clinical manifestations of HCM. The frequency of mutations in each sarcomeric gene may differ between the studies, a likely consequence of the different genetic backgrounds of the populations. Most HCM genetic studies have been based on populations from Europe and Asia, whereas data from African cohorts remains limited.

Keywords: hypertrophic cardiomyopathy, molecular diagnosis, sarcomere, sudden cardiac death

INTRODUCTION

Hypertrophic cardiomyopathy (HCM) is the most common monogenic cardiovascular disorder, affecting one out of every 500 adults (Maron BJ et al. 1995). The disease is defined as abnormal thickening of the left ventricular (LV) myocardium without chamber dilatation and in the absence of any other systemic disease leading to increased afterload excess due to aortic stenosis or hypertension. Hypertrophy is typically asymmetric and sometimes exuberant (Hensley N et al. 2015).

HISTOPATHOLOGY

Major underlying histopathological abnormalities include myofibrillary disarray, in which cardiomyocytes are arranged in a disorganized pattern, and a striking increase in interstitial connective tissue. Replacement fibrosis may be pericellular, patchy, or extensive and is often most prominent in the ventricular septum (Hughes SE. 2004). Dysfunction of the coronary microvasculature together with increased wall thickening leads to luminal narrowing, silent myocardial ischemia, and myocardial injury and fibrosis (Camici PG et al. 2012). Mitral valve abnormalities, including aberrant papillary muscles, abnormal papillary muscle insertion into the anterior mitral leaflet, and enlargement and elongation of mitral leaflets, are extremely common in HCM and are responsible for the development of an abnormal dynamic LV outflow tract (LVOT) gradient. Hypertrophy in HCM most commonly involves the interventricular septum to varying degrees. However, variations do occur: hypertrophy can be concentric, may occur only in the apex or free wall of the LV at the midventricular level, may only affect the outflow tract of the left ventricle, or may include the right ventricular (RV) myocardium (Maron MS et al. 2011).

Genetics

HCM is a disorder due to single gene mutations in germinal cells and thereby inherited in an autosomal dominant Mendelian pattern with variable expressivity and penetrance, meaning that males and females are equally affected and that a mutation in only one of the two copies we all have for every gene is enough to cause the disease. As such, a person carrying the mutation has a 50% chance of passing it to his or her children. The mutation may also arise spontaneously de novo early during embryogenesis rather than being inherited from a parent. This is known as sporadic or spontaneous mutation, which still has a 50% chance of hereditary transmission to the descendants (Maron BJ et al. 2012). Penetrance of LV hypertrophy (LVH) is age dependent. LVH often becomes apparent during adolescence or young adulthood, around the onset of puberty. However, LVH can develop in infancy, early childhood, or late in life (Niimura H et al. 2002). Population studies have shown a significant correlation between LV hypertrophy and age, with 55% penetrance between ages 10–29 versus 95% after age 50 (Ingles J et al. 2013).

Molecular genetic studies have defined HCM as a disease of the sarcomere. The sarcomere is the basic functional unit of muscle structure. It consists of long fibrous proteins responsible for muscular contraction and relaxation. Repeating sarcomere sections form tubular myofibrils, which are essential constituents of tubular muscle cells or myocytes. The sarcomere is formed by contractile myofibrils composed of thick filaments (myosin) and thin filaments (actin) and associated with regulatory proteins which are attached and overlap, allowing muscular contraction (Layland Jand Shah AM. 2006). Proteins involved in maintaining and regulating sarcomere structure and function include myosin binding protein (MyBP)-c, titin, tropomyosin and troponins (C, I, and T) (Solaro RJ. 2010). Numerous mitochondria, responsible for generating adenosine triphosphate for contraction, are scattered between myofibrils (Layland Jand Shah AM. 2006). Contractions of the sarcomere are initiated by calcium binding to troponin C, enabling extensions of the myosin molecules to interact with actin molecules through an adenosine triphosphate-dependent process (Fatkin D and Graham RM. 2002). Electrical excitation of the myocyte results in a high increase in the intracellular calcium concentration, an event called excitation-contraction coupling that initiates further release of calcium from the sarcoplasmic reticulum. Relaxation occurs by lowering the calcium concentration in the myocyte and consecutive detachment from troponin C (Parmacek MS and Solaro RJ. 2004).

The most frequently encountered mutations fall within the genes encoding the β-myosin heavy chain (*MYH7*, 20%–30%, chromosome 14), myosin-binding protein C (MYBPC3; 30%–40%, chromosome 11), cardiac troponin I (*TNNI3*; 7%, chromosome 19), troponin T (*TNNT2;* 10%, chromosome 1), *MYL2* (myosin light chain 2;4%, chromosome 12), *MYL3* (myosin light chain 3; 2%, chromosome 3), and *TPM1* (tropomyosin 1, 1%, chromosome 15) [Table 1]. Mutations in one of these genes are found in approximately 50%-60% of probands (adult and children) with a family history of HCM, and approximately 20%-30% of probands without a family history of HCM (Konno T et al. 2010; Jaafar N et al. 2016). Some patients (2-5%) harbour two mutations in causative sarcomeric genes (either biallelic variants in one gene or heterozygous variants in more than one gene) (Ingles J et al. 2005). These patients exhibit more severe and earlier onset of hypertrophy (Van Driest SL et al. 2004). It has been proposed that one mutation may act as a modifier to the other (Richard P. 2003). Mitochondrial etiologies, though less frequently involved, have also been implicated in HCM (Kuno et al. 2017). Since HCM results from mutations in genes which encode sarcomeric proteins, many questions about cell biology of the cardiac muscle are raised. What is the mechanism by which cardio specific phenotypes result from mutations in sarcomere genes? What intracellular signaling pathways are triggered by the expression of these gene defects? Is the hypertrophic response compensatory or pathologic? The pathogenesis of sarcomeric HCM has been varyingly attributed to increased sarcomeric Ca2+ sensitivity, increased ATPase activity/force, aberrant cross-bridge dynamics leading to complications such as oxidative stress (Lombardi R et al. 2009), and altered sarcomeric phosphorylation (Van Dijk SJ et al. 2009; Hernandez OM et al. 2001; Marston SB. 2011). In HCM, mutations occurring at the level of the sarcomere will ultimately result in inefficient or excessive consumption of adenosine triphosphate and therefore in energy deficiency (Poggesi C and Ho CY. 2014). Mutations affecting the thin-filament regulatory proteins tropomyosin, troponin T, and troponin I all enhance calcium sensitivity by increasing the affinity of troponin C for calcium (Robinson P et al. 2007). Mutations affecting myosin and cMyBP-C also increase this affinity by forming additional cross-bridges between thick and thin filaments. Since troponin is the principal dynamic calcium buffer in the sarcoplasm (Smith GA et al. 2000), the increased affinity should elevate calcium levels during diastole (Kataoka A et al. 2007). Second, sarcomeric mutations increase the energy requirements of myosin ATPase. Since the cross-bridge cycle, which generates the contractile force of the myocyte, accounts for about 70% of the cardiomyocyte's ATP consumption, contractile inefficiency could compromise the energetics of the cardiomyocyte (Ashrafian H et al. 2003). Energy deficiency could reduce the activity of other ATP-consuming processes such as ion pumps (in particular, the sarco-endoplasmic reticulum Ca2+ ATPase [SERCA]), thereby reducing calcium uptake during diastole (Minamisawa S and Ikeda Y. 2006). There is evidence of increased tension-dependent ATP consumption (tension cost) in isolated myofibril preparations (Belus A et al. 2008) and of compromised energetics in mouse models and in patients with cardiomyopathy, including mutation carriers before hypertrophy has developed (Crilley JG et al. 2003). Moreover, other diseases that limit myocardial energy production, including mitochondrial transfer RNA mutations, cause HCM (Ashrafian H et al. 2003).

Ultimately, the effect of a mutation on the contraction of the cardiac muscle will depend on the mutated gene, the location of the mutation within the gene, and consequently on the protein and the abundance of the mutated protein within the myocyte (Maron BJ et al. 2012). Approximately 6% of affected individuals have more than one sarcomere gene DNA variant (either biallelic variants in one gene or heterozygous variants in more than one gene), but a much smaller number will have more than one pathogenic variant (Ingles et al. 2013; Jaafar N et al. 2016).

The absence of sarcomeric gene mutations in the remaining HCM population may be due to shortcomings in current mutation detection methods and strategies, or because patients have disease-causing mutations in genes which encode proteins that are not integral components of the contractile apparatus (Z-disc proteins and calcium handling), such as muscle LIM protein, encoded by *CSRP3*, telethonin, encoded by *TCAP*, vinculin and metavinculin, α-actinin 2, phospholamban encoded by myozenin-2, junctophilin 2 and FLNC encodes for a protein involved in the muscular function of the heart by interacting with the components of sarcolemma and Z-disc [table1]. These variants potentially disrupt processes common to the downstream consequences of myofilament mutations, such as mechano-sensory signaling and calcium handling. Another possible explanation for the low proportion of cases thought to be caused by sarcomere gene mutations is that the HCM population without sarcomeric gene mutations could have one of several diseases that mimic the phenotypic expression of HCM (i.e., phenocopies of the disease: metabolic/infiltrative disease). These phenocopies include various types of metabolic disease (e.g., glycogen storage disease II and III), Anderson–Fabry disease, mitochondrial diseases (e.g., MERRF, MELAS..), syndromes (e.g., Noonan and LEOPARD syndromes), Friedreich's ataxia, and other rare diseases [Table 2]. It is important to recognize the differential phenotypes and/or perform the molecular test to identify these phenocopy diseases, as treatments vary considerably. Both Danon disease and Anderson–Fabry disease can present primarily with cardiac manifestations and mimic HCM caused by sarcomeric mutations; however, these metabolic diseases involve fundamentally different pathological processes and have different clinical courses and require different therapeutic strategies compared to those typically used to treat HCM patients. Danon disease has a severe prognosis that may warrant earlier consideration of a heart transplant (Maron BJ et al. 2009). Anderson–Fabry disease is treated primarily with enzyme replacement (Hoffmann B. 2009). Recent recommendations of the Heart Failure Society of America recommend genetic testing when cardiomyopathy is associated with extra-cardiac manifestations (level of evidence grade A), since many of these HCM phenocopy diseases can be detected by genetic testing (Hershberger RE. 2009).

Molecular Diagnosis

In the last 25 years, the identification of disease-causing mutations in cardiac sarcomere proteins by high-throughput sequencing has opened up the "molecular era" in of understanding of the pathophysiology of inherited cardiomyopathies (Jarcho JA et al. 1989; Priori SG et al. 2003). The use of genetic testing for HCM was initially limited to research laboratories for the purpose of understanding the genetic basis of the disease. Thanks to the availability of newer sequencing technology genetic testing became more widespread in 2003.

New sequencing technologies have led to a striking reduction of costs, by 80-90% for genetic work-up of all cardiomyopathies, and to valuable time-saving. NGS (next generation sequencing) is a promising option for Sanger sequencing, but its clinical utility in analyzing a panel of genes or exomes is based on the ability to enrich or amplify regions of interest with precision (Wooderchak-Donahue et al. 2012).

Table 1. HCM genes

Gene	Locus	Protein	Frequency familial (%)	Frequency sporadic (%)	OMIM	Reference
Myofilament HCM						
MYH7	14q11.2–q12	Beta-myosin heavy chain	30-40	30-40	160760	Van Driest SL et al., 2004
MYBPC3	11p11.2	Cardiac myosin-binding protein C	30-40	30-40	600958	Van Driest SL et al., 2004
TNNT2	1q32	Cardiac troponin T	10-20	10-20	191045	Van Driest SL et al., 2005
TNNI3	19p13.4	Cardiac troponin I	2-5	N.A	191044	Van Driest SL et al., 2005; Kimura A et al., 1997
TPM1	15q22.1	Alpha-tropomyosin	2-5	N.A	191010	Van Driest SL et al., 2005
MYL2	12q23–q24.3	Ventricular regulatory myosin light chain	Rare	Rare	160781	Poetter K et al., 1996
MYL3	3p21.2–p21.3	Ventricular essential myosin light chain	Rare	Rare	160790	Poetter K et al., 1996
ACTC1	15q14	Alpha-cardiacactin	Rare	Rare	102540	Mogensen et al., 1990
TNNC1	3p21.3–p14.3	Cardiac troponin C	Rare	Rare	191040	
TTN	2q24.3	Titin	Rare	Rare	188840	Herman DS et al., 2012
MYH6	14q11.2–q12	Alpha-myosin heavy chain	Rare	Rare	160710	Carniel E et al., 2005
Z-disc HCM						
CSRP3	11p15.1	Muscle LIM protein	N.A	N.A	600824	Knoll R et al., 2002; Geier C et al.,2003
TCAP	17q12–q21.1	Telethonin	Rare	Rare	604488	Hayashi T et al., 2004
VCL	10q22.1–q23	Vinculin/metavinculin	N.A	N.A	193065	Vasile VC et al., 2006
ACTN2	1q42–q43	Alpha-actinin 2	N.A	N.A	102573	Chiu C et al., 2010; Girolami F et al., 2014

Gene	Locus	Protein	Frequency familial (%)	Frequency sporadic (%)	OMIM	Reference
MYOZ2	4q26–q27	Myozenin 2	N.A	N.A	605602	Ruggiero A et al., 2013; Posch MG et al., 2008
NEXN	1p31.1	Nexiline	N.A	N.A	613121	Wang et al., 2010
FLNC	7q32.1	Filamin-C			102565	Valdés-Mas et al., 2014
Calcium-handling						
JPH2	20q12	Junctophilin-2	N.A	N.A	605267	Landstrom AP. 2007 Landstrom AP et al., 2011 a;
PLN	6q22.1	Phospholamban	N.A	N.A	172405	Landstrom AP et al., 2011 b; Maryam Fish et al., 2016
Sarcolemma						
CAV3	3p25.3	Caveolin-3 (M-caveolin)	N.A	N.A	601253	Hayashi T et al., 2004b

OMIM: Online Mendelian Inheritance in Man

Rare: denotes a frequency usually <1%.

N.A: not available

Most laboratories (Harvard Partners, Correlagen, PGxHealth, and GeneDX) provide genetic testing for the most commonly susceptible genes as panel testing for each of the diseases (*MYH7*, *MYH6*, *MYBPC3*, *TNNT2*, *TNNI3*, *TPM1*). Some other laboratories offer a large spectrum of genes for even the rarest forms of each disorder (*MYL2*, *MYL3*, *ACTC*, *TNNC1*, *CSRP3*, *LAMP2*, and *PRKG2*) (Tester DJ and Ackerman MJ. 2011), either of the full protein-encoding region of each gene (whole exome sequencing 'WES') or only the regions of genes where mutations have been shown to reside.

The impact of high-throughput sequencing has markedly increased diagnostic yield. Detection rates of a pathogenic mutation in sporadic and familial HCM cases now range from 40 to 60% (Richard P et al. 2003). However, knowing the underlying HCM genetic mutations still has a limited prognostic relevance as long as genotype-phenotype correlations are not well established. Identifying causative mutations is important in a proband with HCM; both for facilitating pre-symptomatic diagnosis of other family members, clinical surveillance and reproductive advice, and for ascertaining the definite genetic status and diagnosis of HCM. In fact, in the absence of genetic testing, all first-degree subjects who are highly susceptible to HCM should be monitored on average every 12 to 18 months regardless of whether the patient is a child or adult and about every five years by echocardiogram for adults (Gersh BJ et al. 2011). Carriers of the causal mutation should be followed only if the subjects are known to be a definite risk (Gollob MH et al. 2011).

A negative genetic testing provides some reassurance because it may indicate a milder phenotype from a rare variant with better prognosis or a non-genetic etiology (Bos JM et al. 2009; Olivotto I et al. 2008). Mutation-negative family members and their descendants have in fact no risk of developing HCM and do not require further clinical surveillance (Bos JM et al. 2009). If an asymptomatic family member appears to be the carrier of the index case's mutation (genotype positive/phenotype negative), regular cardiac screening must be done by clinical exam, ECG, echocardiography, and Holter monitoring for the rest of their lives because a delayed onset may unexpectedly pose a risk of sudden death in adults and middle-aged individuals who were defined as negative phenotype at an early age. A genetic test result in the absence of clinical manifestations is not an indication that an implantable cardioverter defibrillator (ICD) must be used and there is currently no specific therapy available targeting particular HCM-causing gene mutations.

Although a negative genetic test cannot rule out HCM, a positive genetic test may make it possible to distinguish HCM from exercise-adaptive hypertrophy (athlete's heart) (Bahlmann E et al. 2015) or from HCM phenocopies [Table 2], for which there are definitive and alternative therapies distinct from the HCM treatments available (Robin NH et al. 2007). For example, a positive genetic test in athletes would have an impact on their sports career and might lead to cessation of competitive sport, even in the absence of overt disease (Ho CY. 2010). In this case, mutation-specific genetic testing should be performed on all first-degree family members and appropriate relatives to identify those with unrecognized disease. It has been shown that genetic screening in families with a known mutation is cost-effective, allowing half of the relatives tested to be discharged without the need for clinical investigation or long-term follow-up (Wordsworth S et al. 2010). In addition, it is more sensitive than clinical screening, since ECG or echocardiographic abnormalities may be absent or subtle, or develop later in life.

Reduced penetrance and variable expressivity of inherited cardiomyopathies represent a significant challenge to appropriate diagnosis, pedigree interpretation, and risk stratification of genetic disorders.

Other fields of '-omics,' novel pathways underlying the pathophysiology of cardiac hypertrophy and HCM, have been identified using several new techniques to study large-scale transcriptional changes (Churchill GA. 2002). In fact, microarray tools that allow large numbers of measurements in a single manipulation (thousands of genes simultaneously) provide a snapshot view of gene expression and make it easier to compare expression levels in certain disease states of healthy control subjects. Microarray tools help identify new genes and know about their function and expression levels under different conditions.

Table 2. HCM caused by metabolic/infiltrative disease

Gene	Locus	Protein	Syndrome	Cardiac phenotype	OMIM	Reference
PRKAG2	7q35–q36.36	AMP-activated protein kinase	Wolff-Parkinson-White (WPW)/HCM	Ventricular pre-excitation, supraventricular arrhythmias, progressive conductive disease, abnormal cardiac glycogen storage, and unexplained cardiac hypertrophy.	602743	Zhang BL et al., 2013
LAMP2	Xq24	Lysosome-associated membrane protein 2	Danon's syndrome/WPW	Accumulation of autophagic vacuoles, ventricular preexcitation and rapid disease progression with a nearly universally grave prognosis from life-threatening ventricular arrhythmias and/or progression to end-stage heart failure. Extracardiac manifestations: skeletal myopathy and neurologic and ophthalmologic manifestations including retinal dystrophy.	309060	Arad M et al., 2005 Maron BJ et al. 2009
GLA	Xq22	Alpha-galactosidase A	Fabry’s disease	Unexplained Left Ventricular Hypertrophy (LVH), myocardial fibrosis (mid-myocardial layers), accumulation of glycosphingolipids in the tissues and vasculature, conduction abnormalities, ischemic heart disease. Extracardiac manifestations: severe limb pain, telangiectasia, angiokeratomas, lip thickening, and bulbous nose.	300644	Sachdev B et al., 2002 Song X et al., 2016
GAA	17q25.2–q25.3	Alpha-1,4-glucosidase deficiency	Pompe’s disease	Vacuolar glycogen accumulation leading thickening of the ventricular walls and intraventricular septum (unexplained LVH). Extracardiac manifestations :severe generalized skeletal muscle hypotonia is pronounced in classic infantile form	606800	TuraçaL et al., 2015
AGL	1p21	Amylo-1,6-glucosidase	Glygogen storage disease II and III	Glycogen deposition in cardiac muscle leading thickening of the ventricular walls and intraventricular septum. (unexplained LVH).	610860	Wu XY et al., 2013 Amato AA. 2000

Gene	Locus	Protein	Syndrome	Cardiac phenotype	OMIM	Reference
				Conduction defects. Extracardiac manifestations :muscle weakness, hepatomegaly and hypoglycemia due to liver disease, hyperlipidemia, and growth retardation.		
FXN	9q13	Frataxin	Friedrich's ataxia	Increased iron resulting from reduced mitochondria respiration, decreased cardiac bioenergetics, and LVH. Extracardiac manifestations: neurologic dysfunction, specifically ataxia (incoordination) of all four limbs, and diabetes.	606829	Van den Ouweland AM et al., 2012 Palau F et al., 2001
TAZ	Xq28	Tafazzin (G4.5)	Barth syndrome/ Left Ventricular Non-compaction (LVNC)	cardiomyopathy, neutropenia, skeletal myopathy, growth deficiency, and 3-methylglutaconic aciduria, left ventricular (LV) dilation, hypertrophy, and noncompaction, with varying degrees of congestive heart failure and endocardial fibroelastosis. present at birth and often is cyclic. Biochemical abnormalities: low plasma cholesterol, myopathy	300394	Spencer CT et al., 2006
DTNA	18q12,1	Alpha-dystrobrevin			601239	Bleyl SB et al., 1997
RAF1	3p25.2	V-RAF-1 murine leukemia viral oncogene homolog 1	LEOPARD syndrome (LS)/Noonan's syndrome (NS)	NS: short stature, Developmental delay (DD), mental retardation (MR), characteristic facies, neck webbing, pectus carinatum/excavatum, delayed puberty, cryptorchidism/LS: lentigines, ECG conduction abnormalities, ocular hypertelorism, pulmonic stenosis, abnormal genitalia, growth retardation, sensorineural deafness, skeletal abnormalities, cognitive dysfunction	611553	Passariello Clet al., 2016 Sarkozy A et al., 2003
PTPN11	12q24.13	Protein tyrosine phosphatase non receptor type 11, SHP -2			163950	Qiu W et al., 2014
KRAS	12p12.1	v-Ki-ras2 kirsten rat sarcoma viral oncogene-homolog	Noonan's syndrome	Dysmorphic facial features, cardiac abnormalities, and short stature, among other features. Conduction abnormalities, LVH, valve	609942	Schubbert S et al., 2006

Table 2. (Continued)

Gene	Locus	Protein	Syndrome	Cardiac phenotype	OMIM	Reference
SOS1	2p22-p21	Son of sevenless homolog 1		abnormalities, coronary artery abnormalities, ventricular septal defects. NS-Pulmonary Valve stenosis, atrial septal defects, ventricular septal defects, LVH, persistent ductus arteriosus, conduction defects. Extracardiac manifestations: Electroencephalography (EEG) abnormalities, including bundle branch block, wide set eyes, pulmonary stenosis, abnormal genitalia, missing testicle/ovary, retarded growth, and deafness.	182530	Tartaglia M et al., 2007
ANT1	4q35	Adenine Nucleotide Translocator 1	Progressive external ophthalmoplegia with ragged red fibers	Lactic acidosis, mild myopathy	103220	Palmieri L et al., 2005
MTTK	mtDNA	tRNA Lys	MERRF	Myoclonic epilepsy with ragged red fibers (MERRF), hearing loss	590060	Santorelli F. M et al., 1996
MTATP6	mtDNA	ATP synthase 6	Leigh syndrome	Progressive neurodegeneration	516060	Tatuch Y et al., 1992
MTTL1	mtDNA	tRNALeu-UUR	MELAS	Encephalopathy, lactic acidosis, stroke (MELAS)	590050	Yasukawa T et al., 200
MTTG	mtDNA	tRNAGly	Maternally inherited HCM	Bowel dysmotility	590035	Merante F et al., 1994
MTND1	mtDNA	NADH dehydrogenase, subunit 1	Multisystem mitochondrial diseases	MR, type 2 diabetes	516000	Kirby D. M et al., 2004 DiMauro S and Schon EA. 2003

Abbreviation: OMIM is Online Mendelian Inheritance in Man

Analyzing gene panels with multiple genes involved in HCM implies identifying a large number of variants of uncertain clinical significance (VUS) (Lopes LR et al. 2015).

Other studies have demonstrated the role of miRNAs (micro-ribonucleic acids) in cardiac remodeling and developing hypertrophy disease (van Rooij E et al. 2006) as well as in orchestrating organogenesis and early embryonic patterning processes (Thum T. et al. 2007).

An RNA detection technique (PMAGE) has recently made it possible to identify early transcriptional changes preceding pathological manifestation, including low abundance mRNA (Kim JB et al. 2007).

In the United States, many insurance companies have begun to acknowledge the clinical utility of microarray tools and have implemented favorable reimbursement policies (Maron BJ et al., 1998). Similarly, a Canadian position statement published in 2011 regarding HCM recommends genetic testing of the affected population to permit screening of relatives and treating affected individuals in a timely manner. Effective treatments to prevent sudden cardiac death, such as ICD, do exist. Guidelines have also been drawn up by the Heart Failure Society of America concerning cardiac surveillance and genetic testing in cardiomyopathy (Ingles J et al. 2011) which recommend incorporating clinical genetic testing into routine patient care and highlight the importance of genetic counseling for patients and at-risk family members (Ackerman MJ et al. 2011; Hershberger RE et al. 2009).

Conclusion

Inherited Hypertrophic cardiomyopathy is a disease spread worldwide with reported cases on all continents, affecting people of both sexes and of various racial and ethnic origins. Expanding genetic screening analysis in HCM patients by using NGS technology significantly increases genetic-positive yield, with the added value of detecting other novel variations or discovering new genes susceptible to HCM. Future work should focus on more precise clarification of the pathogenicity of the substantial number of new variants currently known (for which clinical relevance is uncertain) and those that will inevitably be identified by these new molecular techniques.

REFERENCES

Ackerman, MJ; Priori, SG; Willems, S; Berul, C; Brugada, R; Calkins, H; Camm, AJ; et al. "HRS/EHRA Expert Consensus Statement on the State of Genetic Testing for the Channelopathies and Cardiomyopathies." [In English]. *Heart Rhythm*, 8, no. 8 (Aug 2011), 1308-39.

Amato, AA. "Acid Maltase Deficiency and Related Myopathies." *Neurol Clin*, 18, no. 1 (Feb 2000), 151-65

Arad, M; Maron, BJ; Gorham, JM; Johnson, WH; Saul, JP; Perez-Atayde, AR; Spirito, P; et al. "Glycogen Storage Diseases Presenting as Hypertrophic Cardiomyopathy." [In English]. *New England Journal of Medicine*, 352, no. 4 (Jan 27 2005), 362-72.

Ashrafian, H; Redwood, C; Blair, E; Watkins, H. "Hypertrophic Cardiomyopathy: A Paradigm for Myocardial Energy Depletion." [In English]. *Trends in Genetics*, 19, no. 5 (May 2003), 263-68.

Bahlmann, E; Kuck, KH; Nienaber, CA. "Athlete's heart and hypertrophic cardiomyopathy: contribution on clinical and morphologic differentiation". *Dtsch Med Wochenschr*. (July 2015); 140(15):1158-64.

Banerjee, SK; McGaffin, KR; Huang, XYN; Ahmad, F. "Activation of Cardiac Hypertrophic Signaling Pathways in a Transgenic Mouse with the Human Prkag2 Thr400asn Mutation." [In English]. *Biochimica Et Biophysica Acta-Molecular Basis of Disease*, 1802, no. 2 (Feb 2010), 284-91

Belus, A; Piroddi, N; Scellini, B; Tesi, C; Amati, GD; Girolami, F; Yacoub, M; et al. "The Familial Hypertrophic Cardiomyopathy-Associated Myosin Mutation R403q Accelerates Tension Generation and Relaxation of Human Cardiac Myofibrils." [In English]. *Journal of Physiology-London*, 586, no. 15 (Aug 1 2008), 3639-44.

Bleyl, SB; Mumford, BR; Thompson, V; Carey, JC; Pysher, TJ; Chin, TK; Ward, K. "Neonatal, Lethal Noncompaction of the Left Ventricular Myocardium Is Allelic with Barth Syndrome." [In English]. *American Journal of Human Genetics*, 61, no. 4 (Oct 1997), 868-72.

Bos, JM; Towbin, JA; Ackerman, MJ. "Diagnostic, Prognostic, and Therapeutic Implications of Genetic Testing for Hypertrophic Cardiomyopathy." [In English]. *Journal of the American College of Cardiology*, 54, no. 3 (Jul 14 2009), 201-11.

Camici, PG; Olivotto, I; Rimoldi, OE. "The Coronary Circulation and Blood Flow in Left Ventricular Hypertrophy." [In English]. *Journal of Molecular and Cellular Cardiology*, 52, no. 4 (Apr 2012), 857-64.

Carniel, E; Taylor, MRG; Sinagra, G; Di Lenarda, A; Ku, L; Fain, PR; Boucek, MM;et al. "Alpha-Myosin Heavy Chain - a Sarcomeric Gene Associated with Dilated and Hypertrophic Phenotypes of Cardiomyopathy." [In English]. *Circulation*,112, no. 1 (Jul 5 2005), 54-59.

Chiu, C; Bagnall, RD; Ingles, J; Yeates, L; Kennerson, M; Donald, JA; Jormakka, M; Lind, JM; Semsarian, C. "Mutations in Alpha-Actinin-2 Cause Hypertrophic Cardiomyopathy a Genome-Wide Analysis." [In English]. *Journal of the American College of Cardiology*, 55, no. 11 (Mar 16 2010), 1127-35.

Churchill, GA. "Fundamentals of Experimental Design for Cdna Microarrays." *Nat Genet*, 32, Suppl (Dec 2002), 490-5.

Crilley, JG; Boehm, EA; Blair, E; Rajagopalan, B; Blamire, AM; Styles, P; McKenna, WJ;et al. "Hypertrophic Cardiomyopathy Due to Sarcomeric Gene Mutations Is Characterized by Impaired Energy Metabolism Irrespective of the Degree of Hypertrophy." *J Am Coll Cardiol*, 41, no. 10 (May 21 2003), 1776-82.

DiMauro, S; Schon, EA. "Mitochondrial Respiratory-Chain Diseases." *N Engl J Med*, 348, no. 26 (Jun 26 2003), 2656-68.

Fatkin, D; Graham, RM. "Molecular Mechanisms of Inherited Cardiomyopathies." *Physiol Rev*, 82, no. 4 (Oct 2002), 945-80.

Fish, M; Shaboodien, G; Kraus, S; Sliwa, K; Seidman, CE; Burke, MA; Crotti, L; Schwartz, PJ; Mayosi, BM. "Mutation Analysis of the

Phospholamban Gene in 315 South Africans with Dilated, Hypertrophic, Peripartum and Arrhythmogenic Right Ventricular Cardiomyopathies." *Sci Rep*,6, (Feb 26 2016), 22235.

Geier, C; Perrot, A; Ozcelik, C; Binner, P; Counsell, D; Hoffmann, K; Pilz, B;et al. "Mutations in the Human Muscle Lim Protein Gene in Families with Hypertrophic Cardiomyopathy." *Circulation*, 107, no. 10 (Mar 18 2003), 1390-5.

Gersh, BJ; Maron, BJ; Bonow, RO; Dearani, JA; Fifer, MA; Link, MS; Naidu,SS;et al. "2011 Accf/Aha Guideline for the Diagnosis and Treatment of Hypertrophic Cardiomyopathy: A Report of the American College of Cardiology Foundation/American Heart Association Task Force on Practice Guidelines. Developed in Collaboration with the American Association for Thoracic Surgery, American Society of Echocardiography, American Society of Nuclear Cardiology, Heart Failure Society of America, Heart Rhythm Society, Society for Cardiovascular Angiography and Interventions, and Society of Thoracic Surgeons." *J Am Coll Cardiol*, 58, no. 25 (Dec 13 2011), e212-60.

Girolami, F; Iascone, M; Tomberli, B; Bardi, S; Benelli, M; Marseglia, G; Pescucci, C;et al."Novel Alpha-Actinin 2 Variant Associated with Familial Hypertrophic Cardiomyopathy and Juvenile Atrial Arrhythmias: A Massively Parallel Sequencing Study." *Circ Cardiovasc Genet*, 7, no. 6 (Dec 2014), 741-50.

Gollob, MH; Blier, L; Brugada, R; Champagne, J; Chauhan, V; Connors, S; Gardner, M;et al. "Recommendations for the Use of Genetic Testing in the Clinical Evaluation of Inherited Cardiac Arrhythmias Associated with Sudden Cardiac Death: Canadian Cardiovascular Society/Canadian Heart Rhythm Society Joint Position Paper." *Can J Cardiol*, 27, no. 2 (Mar-Apr 2011), 232-45.

Hayashi, T; Arimura, T; Itoh-Satoh, M; Ueda, K; Hohda, S; Inagaki, N; Takahashi, M; et al. "Tcap Gene Mutations in Hypertrophic Cardiomyopathy and Dilated Cardiomyopathy." *J Am Coll Cardiol*,44, no. 11 (Dec 07 2004), 2192-201.

Hayashi, T; Arimura, T; Ueda, K; Shibata, H; Hohda, S; Takahashi, M; Hori, H: et al. "Identification and Functional Analysis of a Caveolin-3 Mutation Associated with Familial Hypertrophic Cardiomyopathy." *Biochem Biophys Res Commun*, 313, no. 1 (Jan 02 2004), 178-84.

Hensley, N; Dietrich, J; Nyhan, D; Mitter, N; Yee, MS; Brady, M. "Hypertrophic Cardiomyopathy: A Review." *Anesth Analg*, 20, no. 3 (Mar 2015), 554-69.

Herman, DS; Lam, L; Taylor, MR; Wang, L; Teekakirikul, P; Christodoulou, D; Conner, L; et al. "Truncations of Titin Causing Dilated Cardiomyopathy." *N Engl J Med*, 366, no. 7 (Feb 16 2012), 619-28.

Hernandez, OM; Housmans, PR; Potter, JD. "Invited Review: Pathophysiology of Cardiac Muscle Contraction and Relaxation as a Result of Alterations in Thin Filament Regulation." *J Appl Physiol (1985)*, 90, no. 3 (Mar 2001), 1125-36.

Hershberger, RE; Cowan, J; Morales, A; Siegfried, JD. "Progress with Genetic Cardiomyopathies: Screening, Counseling, and Testing in Dilated, Hypertrophic, and Arrhythmogenic Right Ventricular Dysplasia/Cardiomyopathy." *Circ Heart Fail*, 2, no. 3 (May 2009), 253-61.

Hershberger, RE; Lindenfeld, J; Mestroni, L; Seidman, CE; Taylor, MR; Towbin, JA. America Heart Failure Society of. "Genetic Evaluation of Cardiomyopathy--a Heart Failure Society of America Practice Guideline." *J Card Fail*, 15, no. 2 (Mar 2009), 83-97.

Ho, CY. "Genetics and Clinical Destiny: Improving Care in Hypertrophic Cardiomyopathy." *Circulation*, 122, no. 23 (Dec 07 2010), 2430-40, discussion 40.

Hoffmann, B. "Fabry Disease: Recent Advances in Pathology, Diagnosis, Treatment and Monitoring." *Orphanet J Rare Dis*, 4 (Oct 11 2009), 21.

Hughes, SE. "The Pathology of Hypertrophic Cardiomyopathy." *Histopathology*, 44, no. 5 (May 2004), 412-27.

Ingles, J; Doolan, A; Chiu, C; Seidman, J; Seidman, C; Semsarian, C. "Compound and Double Mutations in Patients with Hypertrophic

Cardiomyopathy: Implications for Genetic Testing and Counselling." *J Med Genet*, 42, no. 10 (Oct 2005), e59.

Ingles, J; Sarina, T; Yeates, L; Hunt, L; Macciocca, I; McCormack, L; Winship, I;et al. "Clinical Predictors of Genetic Testing Outcomes in Hypertrophic Cardiomyopathy." *Genet Med*, 15, no. 12 (Dec 2013), 972-7.

Ingles, J; Zodgekar, PR; Yeates, L; Macciocca, I; Semsarian, C; Fatkin, D. Csanz Cardiac Genetic Diseases Council Writing Group. "Guidelines for Genetic Testing of Inherited Cardiac Disorders." *Heart Lung Circ*, 20, no. 11 (Nov 2011), 681-7.

Jaafar, Nawel; Go´mez, Juan; Kammoun, Ikram; Zairi, Ihsen; Ben, Amara Wael; Kachboura, Salem; et al. Spectrum of Mutations in Hypertrophic Cardiomyopathy Genes Among Tunisian Patients. *Genet Test Mol Biomarkers*., 2016 Nov, 20(11), 674-679.

Jarcho, JA; McKenna, W; Pare, JA; Solomon, SD; Holcombe, RF; Dickie, S; Levi, T; et al. "Mapping a Gene for Familial Hypertrophic Cardiomyopathy to Chromosome 14q1." *N Engl J Med*, 321, no. 20 (Nov 16 1989), 1372-8.

Kataoka, A; Hemmer, C; Chase, PB. "Computational Simulation of Hypertrophic Cardiomyopathy Mutations in Troponin I: Influence of Increased Myofilament Calcium Sensitivity on Isometric Force, Atpase and [Ca2+]I." *J Biomech*, 40, no. 9 (2007), 2044-52.

Kim, JB; Porreca, GJ; Song, L; Greenway, SC; Gorham, JM; Church, GM; Seidman, CE; Seidman, JG. "Polony Multiplex Analysis of Gene Expression (Pmage) in Mouse Hypertrophic Cardiomyopathy." *Science*, 316, no. 5830 (Jun 08 2007), 1481-4.

Kimura, A; Harada, H; Park, JE; Nishi, H; Satoh, M; Takahashi, M; Hiroi,S;et al. "Mutations in the Cardiac Troponin I Gene Associated with Hypertrophic Cardiomyopathy." *Nat Genet*, 16, no. 4 (Aug 1997), 379-82.

Kirby, DM; McFarland, R; Ohtake, A; Dunning, C; Ryan, MT; Wilson, C; Ketteridge, D; et al. "Mutations of the Mitochondrial Nd1 Gene as a Cause of Melas." *J Med Genet*, 41, no. 10 (Oct 2004), 784-9.

Knöll, Ralph; Masahiko, Hoshijima; Kenneth, R Chien. "Muscle Lim Protein in Heart Failure." *Experimental & Clinical Cardiology*, 7, no. 2-3 (2002), 104.

Konno, T; Chang, S; Seidman, JG; Seidman, CE. "Genetics of Hypertrophic Cardiomyopathy." *Curr Opin Cardiol*, 25, no. 3 (May 2010), 205-9.

Kuno, T; Imaeda, S; Asakawa, Y; Nakamura, H; Takemura, G; Asahara, D; Kanamori, A; Kabutoya, T; Numasawa, Y. "Mitochondrial Cardiomyopathy Presenting as Dilated Phase of Hypertrophic Cardiomyopathy Diagnosed with Histological and Genetic Analyses." *Case Rep Cardiol*, 2017 (2017), 9473917.

Landstrom, AP; Adekola, BA; Bos, JM; Ommen, SR; Ackerman, MJ. "Pln-Encoded Phospholamban Mutation in a Large Cohort of Hypertrophic Cardiomyopathy Cases: Summary of the Literature and Implications for Genetic Testing." *Am Heart J*, 161, no. 1 (Jan 2011), 165-71.

Landstrom, AP; Kellen, CA; Dixit, SS; van Oort, RJ; Garbino, A; Weisleder, N; Ma, J; Wehrens, XH; Ackerman, MJ. "Junctophilin-2 Expression Silencing Causes Cardiocyte Hypertrophy and Abnormal Intracellular Calcium-Handling." *Circ Heart Fail*, 4, no. 2 (Mar 2011), 214-23.

Landstrom, AP; Weisleder, N; Batalden, KB; Bos, JM; Tester, DJ; Ommen, SR; Wehrens, XH., et al. "Mutations in Jph2-Encoded Junctophilin-2 Associated with Hypertrophic Cardiomyopathy in Humans." *J Mol Cell Cardiol*, 42, no. 6 (Jun 2007), 1026-35.

Layland, J; Shah, AM. "Biochemistry and Physiology of Cardiac Muscle." *Medicine*, 34, no. 5 (2006/05/01/ 2006), 169-72.

Lombardi, R; Rodriguez, G; Chen, SN; Ripplinger, CM; Li, W; Chen, J; Willerson, JT;et al. "Resolution of Established Cardiac Hypertrophy and Fibrosis and Prevention of Systolic Dysfunction in a Transgenic Rabbit Model of Human Cardiomyopathy through Thiol-Sensitive Mechanisms." *Circulation*, 119, no. 10 (Mar 17 2009), 1398-407.

Lopes, LR; Murphy, C; Syrris, P; Dalageorgou, C; McKenna, WJ; Elliott, PM; Plagnol, V. "Use of High-Throughput Targeted Exome-Sequencing to Screen for Copy Number Variation in Hypertrophic Cardiomyopathy." *Eur J Med Genet*, 58, no. 11 (Nov 2015), 611-6.

Maron, BJ; Gardin, JM; Flack, JM; Gidding, SS; Kurosaki, TT; Bild, DE. "Prevalence of Hypertrophic Cardiomyopathy in a General Population of Young Adults. Echocardiographic Analysis of 4111 Subjects in the Cardia Study. Coronary Artery Risk Development in (Young) Adults." *Circulation*, 92, no. 4 (Aug 15 1995), 785-9.

Maron, BJ; Maron, MS; Semsarian, C. "Genetics of Hypertrophic Cardiomyopathy after 20 Years: Clinical Perspectives." *J Am Coll Cardiol*, 60, no. 8 (Aug 21 2012), 705-15.

Maron, BJ; Moller, JH; Seidman, CE; Vincent, GM; Dietz, HC; Moss, AJ; Towbin, JA;et al. "Impact of Laboratory Molecular Diagnosis on Contemporary Diagnostic Criteria for Genetically Transmitted Cardiovascular Diseases: Hypertrophic Cardiomyopathy, Long-Qt Syndrome, and Marfan Syndrome: A Statement for Healthcare Professionals from the Councils on Clinical Cardiology, Cardiovascular Disease in the Young, and Basic Science, American Heart Association." *Circulation*, 98, no. 14 (Oct 06 1998), 1460-71.

Maron, BJ; Roberts, WC; Arad, M; Haas, TS; Spirito, P; Wright, GB; Almquist, AK., et al. "Clinical Outcome and Phenotypic Expression in Lamp2 Cardiomyopathy." *JAMA*, 301, no. 12 (Mar 25 2009), 1253-9.

Maron, MS; Olivotto, I; Harrigan, C; Appelbaum, E; Gibson, CM; Lesser, JR; Haas, TS; et al. "Mitral Valve Abnormalities Identified by Cardiovascular Magnetic Resonance Represent a Primary Phenotypic Expression of Hypertrophic Cardiomyopathy." *Circulation*, 124, no. 1 (Jul 05 2011), 40-7.

Marston, SB. "How Do Mutations in Contractile Proteins Cause the Primary Familial Cardiomyopathies?". *J Cardiovasc Transl Res*, 4, no. 3 (Jun 2011), 245-55.

Merante, F; Tein, I; Benson, L; Robinson, BH. "Maternally Inherited Hypertrophic Cardiomyopathy Due to a Novel T-to-C Transition at

Nucleotide 9997 in the Mitochondrial Trna(Glycine) Gene." *Am J Hum Genet*, 55, no. 3 (Sep 1994), 437-46.

Minamisawa, S; Ikeda, Y. "Sarcoplasmic Reticulum Function and Heart Failure: A Novel Therapeutic Target for Heart Failure." *Clin Calcium*, 16, no. 1 (Jan 2006), 37-44.

Mogensen, J; Klausen, IC; Pedersen, AK; Egeblad, H; Bross, P; Kruse, TA; Gregersen, N; et al. "Alpha-Cardiac Actin Is a Novel Disease Gene in Familial Hypertrophic Cardiomyopathy." *J Clin Invest*, 103, no. 10 (May 15 1999), R39-43.

Niimura, H; Patton, KK; McKenna, WJ; Soults, J; Maron, BJ; Seidman, JG; Seidman, CE. "Sarcomere Protein Gene Mutations in Hypertrophic Cardiomyopathy of the Elderly." *Circulation*, 105, no. 4 (Jan 29 2002), 446-51.

Olivotto, I; Girolami, F; Ackerman, MJ; Nistri, S; Bos, JM; Zachara, E; Ommen, SR; et al. "Myofilament Protein Gene Mutation Screening and Outcome of Patients with Hypertrophic Cardiomyopathy." *Mayo Clin Proc*, 83, no. 6 (Jun 2008), 630-8.

Palau, F. "Friedreich's Ataxia and Frataxin: Molecular Genetics, Evolution and Pathogenesis (Review)." *Int J Mol Med*, 7, no. 6 (Jun 2001), 581-9.

Palmieri, L; Alberio, S; Pisano, I; Lodi, T; Meznaric-Petrusa, M; Zidar, J; Santoro, A; et al. "Complete Loss-of-Function of the Heart/Muscle-Specific Adenine Nucleotide Translocator Is Associated with Mitochondrial Myopathy and Cardiomyopathy." *Hum Mol Genet*, 14, no. 20 (Oct 15 2005), 3079-88.

Parmacek, MS; Solaro, RJ. "Biology of the Troponin Complex in Cardiac Myocytes." *Prog Cardiovasc Dis*, 47, no. 3 (Nov-Dec 2004), 159-76.

Passariello, CL; Martinez, EC; Thakur, H; Cesareo, M; Li, J; Kapiloff, MS. "Rsk3 Is Required for Concentric Myocyte Hypertrophy in an Activated Raf1 Model for Noonan Syndrome." *J Mol Cell Cardiol*, 93 (Apr 2016), 98-105.

Poetter, K; Jiang, H; Hassanzadeh, S; Master, SR; Chang, A; Dalakas, MC; Rayment, I; et al. "Mutations in Either the Essential or Regulatory Light Chains of Myosin Are Associated with a Rare Myopathy in

Human Heart and Skeletal Muscle." *Nat Genet*, 13, no. 1 (May 1996), 63-9.

Poggesi, C; Ho, CY. "Muscle Dysfunction in Hypertrophic Cardiomyopathy: What Is Needed to Move to Translation?". *J Muscle Res Cell Motil*, 35, no. 1 (Feb 2014), 37-45.

Posch, MG; Thiemann, L; Tomasov, P; Veselka, J; Cardim, N; Garcia-Castro, M; Coto, E;et al. "Sequence Analysis of Myozenin 2 in 438 European Patients with Familial Hypertrophic Cardiomyopathy." *Med Sci Monit*, 14, no. 7 (Jul 2008), CR372-4.

Priori, S; Rivolta, I; Napolitano, C. "Genetics of Long Qt, Brugada, and Other Channelopathies". In D.P. Zipes, & J. Jalife (a cura di), Cardiac Electrophysiology. From Cell to Bedside 4th edition. Philadelphia: American heart association, (2004).

Qiu, W; Wang, X; Romanov, V; Hutchinson, A; Lin, A; Ruzanov, M; Battaile, KP; et al. "Structural Insights into Noonan/Leopard Syndrome-Related Mutants of Protein-Tyrosine Phosphatase Shp2 (Ptpn11)." *BMC Struct Biol*, 14 (Mar 14 2014), 10.

Richard, P; Charron, P; Carrier, L; Ledeuil, C; Cheav, T; Pichereau, C; Benaiche,A;et al. "Hypertrophic Cardiomyopathy: Distribution of Disease Genes, Spectrum of Mutations, and Implications for a Molecular Diagnosis Strategy." *Circulation*, 107, no. 17 (May 06 2003), 2227-32.

Robin, NH; Tabereaux, PB; Benza, R; Korf, BR. "Genetic Testing in Cardiovascular Disease." *J Am Coll Cardiol*, 50, no. 8 (Aug 21 2007), 727-37.

Robinson, P; Griffiths, PJ; Watkins, H; Redwood, CS. "Dilated and Hypertrophic Cardiomyopathy Mutations in Troponin and Alpha-Tropomyosin Have Opposing Effects on the Calcium Affinity of Cardiac Thin Filaments." *Circ Res*, 101, no. 12 (Dec 07 2007), 1266-73.

Sachdev, B; Takenaka, T; Teraguchi, H; Tei, C; Lee, P; McKenna, WJ; Elliott, PM. "Prevalence of Anderson-Fabry Disease in Male Patients with Late Onset Hypertrophic Cardiomyopathy." *Circulation*, 105, no. 12 (Mar 26 2002), 1407-11.

Santorelli, FM; Mak, SC; El-Schahawi, M; Casali, C; Shanske, S; Baram, TZ; Madrid, RE; DiMauro, S. "Maternally Inherited Cardiomyopathy and Hearing Loss Associated with a Novel Mutation in the Mitochondrial Trna(Lys) Gene (G8363a)." *Am J Hum Genet*, 58, no. 5 (May 1996), 933-9.

Sarkozy, A; Conti, E; Seripa, D; Digilio, MC; Grifone, N; Tandoi, C; Fazio, VM; et al. "Correlation between Ptpn11 Gene Mutations and Congenital Heart Defects in Noonan and Leopard Syndromes." *J Med Genet*, 40, no. 9 (Sep 2003), 704-8.

Schubbert, S; Zenker, M; Rowe, SL; Boll, S; Klein, C; Bollag, G; van der Burgt, I; et al. "Germline Kras Mutations Cause Noonan Syndrome." *Nat Genet*, 38, no. 3 (Mar 2006), 331-6.

Smith, GA; Dixon, HB; Kirschenlohr, HL; Grace, AA; Metcalfe, JC; Vandenberg, JI. "Ca2+ Buffering in the Heart: Ca2+ Binding to and Activation of Cardiac Myofibrils." *Biochem J*, 346, Pt 2 (Mar 01 2000), 393-402.

Solaro, RJ. "Sarcomere Control Mechanisms and the Dynamics of the Cardiac Cycle." *J Biomed Biotechnol*, 2010 (2010), 105648.

Song, X; Xue, S; Zhao, J; Wu, J. "Screening for Fabry's Disease in Young Patients with Ischemic Stroke in a Chinese Population." *Int J Neurosci*, 127, no. 4 (Apr 2017), 350-55.

Spencer, CT; Bryant, RM; Day, J; Gonzalez, IL; Colan, SD; Thompson, WR; Berthy, J; Redfearn, SP; Byrne, BJ. "Cardiac and Clinical Phenotype in Barth Syndrome." *Pediatrics*, 118, no. 2 (Aug 2006), e337-46.

Tartaglia, M; Kalidas, K; Shaw, A; Song, X; Musat, DL; van der Burgt, I; Brunner, HG; et al. "Ptpn11 Mutations in Noonan Syndrome: Molecular Spectrum, Genotype-Phenotype Correlation, and Phenotypic Heterogeneity." *Am J Hum Genet*, 70, no. 6 (Jun 2002), 1555-63.

Tartaglia, M; Pennacchio, LA; Zhao, C; Yadav, KK; Fodale, V; Sarkozy, A; Pandit, B; et al. "Gain-of-Function Sos1 Mutations Cause a Distinctive Form of Noonan Syndrome." *Nat Genet*, 39, no. 1 (Jan 2007), 75-9.

Tatuch, Y; Christodoulou, J; Feigenbaum, A; Clarke, JT; Wherret, J; Smith, C; Rudd, N; Petrova-Benedict, R; Robinson, B. H. "Heteroplasmic Mtdna Mutation (T----G) at 8993 Can Cause Leigh Disease When the Percentage of Abnormal Mtdna Is High." *Am J Hum Genet*, 50, no. 4 (Apr 1992), 852-8.

Tester, DJ; Ackerman, MJ. "Genetic Testing for Potentially Lethal, Highly Treatable Inherited Cardiomyopathies/Channelopathies in Clinical Practice." *Circulation*, 123, no. 9 (Mar 08 2011), 1021-37.

Thum, T; Galuppo, P; Wolf, C; Fiedler, J; Kneitz, S; van Laake, LW; Doevendans, PA;et al. "Micrornas in the Human Heart: A Clue to Fetal Gene Reprogramming in Heart Failure." *Circulation*, 116, no. 3 (Jul 17 2007), 258-67.

Turaca, LT; de Faria, DO; Kyosen, SO; Teixeira, VD; Motta, FL; Pessoa, JG; Silva, E; Rodrigues, M; et al. "Novel Gaa Mutations in Patients with Pompe Disease." *Gene*, 561, no. 1 (Apr 25 2015), 124-31.

Valdés-Mas, R; Gutiérrez-Fernandez, A; Gómez, J; et al. (2014). "Mutations in filamin C cause a new form of familial hypertrophic cardiomyopathy". *Nat Commun*, 5, 5326

Van den Ouweland, AM; van Minkelen, R; Bolman, GM; Wouters, CH; Becht-Noordermeer, C; Deelen, WH; Deelen-Manders, JM; et al. "Complete Fxn Deletion in a Patient with Friedreich's Ataxia." *Genet Test Mol Biomarkers*, 16, no. 9 (Sep 2012), 1015-8.

Van Dijk, SJ; Dooijes, D; dos Remedios, C; Michels, M; Lamers, JM; Winegrad, S; Schlossarek, S; et al. "Cardiac Myosin-Binding Protein C Mutations and Hypertrophic Cardiomyopathy: Haploinsufficiency, Deranged Phosphorylation, and Cardiomyocyte Dysfunction." *Circulation*, 119, no. 11 (Mar 24 2009), 1473-83.

Van Driest, SL; Ommen, SR; Tajik, AJ; Gersh, BJ; Ackerman, MJ. "Yield of Genetic Testing in Hypertrophic Cardiomyopathy." *Mayo Clin Proc*, 80, no. 6 (Jun 2005), 739-44.

Van Driest, SL; Vasile, VC; Ommen, SR; Will, ML; Tajik, AJ; Gersh, BJ; Ackerman, MJ. "Myosin Binding Protein C Mutations and Compound Heterozygosity in Hypertrophic Cardiomyopathy." *J Am Coll Cardiol*, 44, no. 9 (Nov 02 2004), 1903-10.

Van Rooij, E; Sutherland, LB; Liu, N; Williams, AH; McAnally, J; Gerard, RD; Richardson, JA; Olson, EN. "A Signature Pattern of Stress-Responsive Micrornas That Can Evoke Cardiac Hypertrophy and Heart Failure." *Proc Natl Acad Sci USA*, 103, no. 48 (Nov 28 2006), 18255-60.

Vasile, VC; Will, ML; Ommen, SR Edwards, WD; Olson, TM; Ackerman, MJ. "Identification of a Metavinculin Missense Mutation, R975w, Associated with Both Hypertrophic and Dilated Cardiomyopathy." *Mol Genet Metab*, 87, no. 2 (Feb 2006), 169-74.

In: Hypertrophic Cardiomyopathy
Editor: Ikram Kammoun
ISBN: 978-1-53613-003-4

Chapter 2

FOCUS ON DIAGNOSIS IN HYPERTROPHIC CARDIOMYOPATHY

Leila Abid**, MD and Salma Charfeddine, MD
Department of cardiology, Sfax University, Sfax, Tunisia

ABSTRACT

Hypertrophic cardiomyopathy (HCM) is a genetic disorder characterized by left ventricular hypertrophy unexplained by secondary causes and a non-dilated left ventricle (LV) with preserved or increased ejection fraction. It is commonly asymmetrical with the most severe hypertrophy involving the interventricular septum. Left ventricular outflow tract obstruction is present at rest in about one third of patients and can be provoked in another third. HCM is an important cause of sudden cardiac death, particularly in adolescents and young adults. A diagnosis of HCM is most often established with noninvasive cardiac imaging, including echocardiography and/or cardiac magnetic resonance imaging.

Keywords: hypertrophic cardiomyopathy, diagnosis, echocardiography, cardiac magnetic resonance

* Corresponding author: leilaabidt@yahoo.fr.

Introduction

Hypertrophic Cardiomyopathy (HCM) is a common genetic cardiovascular disease (Gersh et al. 2011). HCM is a disease state characterized by unexplained, marked and asymmetric left ventricular (LV) hypertrophy associated with non-dilated ventricular chambers in the absence of another cardiac or systemic disease capable of producing the magnitude of hypertrophy evident in a given patient (Elliott et al. 2014). In an adult, HCM is defined by a wall thickness ≥15 mm in one or more LV myocardial segments—as measured by any imaging technique (echocardiography, cardiac magnetic resonance imaging (CMR) or computed tomography (CT))—that is not explained solely by loading conditions. Genetic and non-genetic disorders can present with lesser degrees of wall thickening (13–14 mm); in these cases, diagnosis of HCM requires evaluation of other features including family history, non-cardiac symptoms and signs, electrocardiogram (ECG) abnormalities, laboratory tests and multi-modality cardiac imaging (Elliott et al. 2014).

The following topics are detailed in this chapter:

- History
- Physical examination
- Electrocardiography
- Echocardiography
- Cardiovascular magnetic resonance imaging
- Cardiac computerized tomography
- Laboratory tests
- Genetic testing

History

Most patients with HCM are asymptomatic but some develop symptoms, often many years after the appearance of electrocardiographic or echocardiographic evidence of LVH.

Chest Pain

Many patients complain of angina or atypical chest pain at rest or on exertion. The causes of chest pain include myocardial ischemia due to microvascular dysfunction, increased LV wall stress and LV outflow tract obstruction (LVOTO). Congenital coronary artery anomalies, including tunnelled left anterior descending artery or atherosclerotic coronary artery disease, may also be responsible (Sorajja et al. 2003). Systolic compression of epicardial and intramural vessels is also very common. Pain may also be precipitated by large meals or alcohol (Gilligan et al. 1996, Feiner et al. 2013, Paz et al. 1996).

Dyspnea

Dyspnea is the most common presenting symptom. It is largely a consequence of elevated LV diastolic filling pressures (and transmission of those elevated pressures back into pulmonary circulation). The elevated LV filling pressures are principally caused by impaired diastolic compliance as a result of marked hypertrophy of the ventricle.

Syncope and/or Presyncope

Syncope during exertion, or immediately following palpitation or chest pain, suggests a cardiac mechanism (Moya et al. 2009). Provocable obstruction should be excluded when patients experience recurrent effort syncope in similar circumstances—for example, when hurrying up stairs or straining (Shah et al. 2008). Ventricular arrhythmias are an uncommon cause of syncope, but should be suspected after an unheralded episode, particularly when occurring at rest or after minimal exertion.

Palpitations

Many patients complain of palpitations, caused by symptomatic cardiac contractions and ventricular ectopy (Coats et al. 2013). A sustained episode of palpitation lasting for more than a few minutes is often caused by supraventricular arrhythmia (Gimeno et al. 2009).

Sudden Cardiac Death

This is the most devastating presenting manifestation of HCM. It has the highest incidence in preadolescent and adolescent children and is particularly related to extreme exertion. Sudden death is caused in most cases by ventricular fibrillation. Many of these cases degenerate into ventricular fibrillation from rapid atrial arrhythmias, such as fibrillation, supraventricular tachycardia, or Wolff-Parkinson-White syndrome, while others result from ventricular tachycardia and low cardiac output hemodynamic collapse.

Physical Examination

In HCM, cardiovascular examination is often normal. But, in patients with LV outflow tract obstruction (LVOTO), a number of typical features may be identified including a rapid up-and-down stroke to the arterial pulse and an ejection systolic murmur at the left sternal edge that radiates to the right upper sternal edge and apex. The intensity of the murmur is increased by manoeuvres that reduce ventricular preload or afterload, such as standing up from a squatting position and forceful attempted exhalation against a closed airway (Valsalva manoeuvre). Most patients with LVOTO also have signs of mitral regurgitation (Elliott et al. 2014).

RESTING AND AMBULATORY ELECTROCARDIOGRAPHY (ECG)

The standard 12-lead ECG can be normal at presentation (6% of patients in referral cohort studies) but generally shows a variable combination of LVH, ST- and T-wave abnormalities, and pathological Q-waves (McLeod et al. 2009).

Giant negative T wave inversion (>10 mm) in the precordial and/or inferolateral leads suggests involvement of the LV apex (Figure 1).

Abnormally deep Q waves ≥25% of the R wave in the inferolateral leads, usually with a positive T wave, are associated with an asymmetrical distribution of LVH.

Q waves of abnormal duration (≥40 ms) are associated with areas of fibrosis.

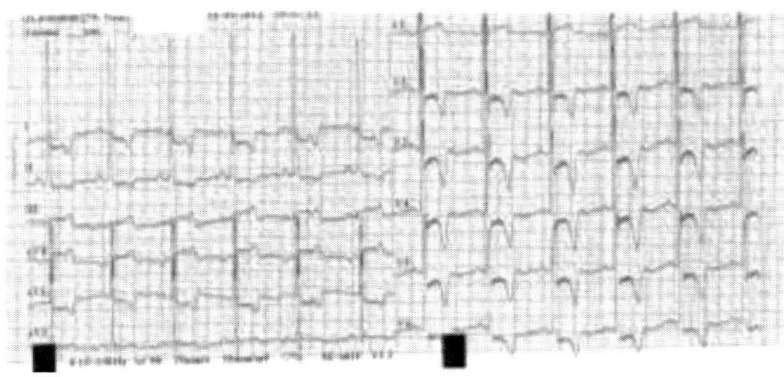

Figure 1. Electrocardiogram showing giant negative T wave inversion (>10 mm) in the precordial and inferolateral leads suggests involvement of the left ventricle apex.

Some patients with apical or distal hypertrophy develop small apical aneurysms, sometimes associated with myocardial scarring. These may only be detectable on CMR, ventriculography or contrast echo, and are occasionally associated with ST elevation in the lateral chest leads.

An ECG is recommended at the first clinic visit for all individuals with known or suspected HCM and should be repeated whenever there is a change in symptoms in patients with an established diagnosis. The ECG is also a sensitive—though non-specific—early marker of disease in relatives (Charron et al. 2003).

The frequency of arrhythmias detected during ambulatory electrocardiographic monitoring is age-related. Asymptomatic non-sustained ventricular tachycardia (NSVT), at a rate between 120 and 200 beats per minute (bpm), occurs in 25% of adults with HCM (Monserrat et al. 2003). Paroxysmal supraventricular arrhythmias occur during ambulatory electrocardiographic monitoring in up to 38% of patients (Adabag et al. 2005). Ambulatory ECG monitoring is recommended at the initial clinical assessment to assess the risk of sudden cardiac death and stroke.

ECHOCARDIOGRAPHY

In order to establish the diagnosis of HCM, a systematic echocardiography approach is necessary. The echocardiography should include:

- Confirming LV hypertrophy
- Assessment of LVOT obstruction
- Systolic anterior motion - SAM
- Assessment of systolic and diastolic LV function and left atrial size

Additional novel echocardiographic modalities allow better understanding of subclinical LV damage. Transthoracic echocardiography is recommended for screening patients with HCM family members.

Confirming Left Ventricular Hypertrophy

Hypertrophy preferentially involves the interventricular septum in the basal LV segments but often extends into the lateral wall, posterior septum and LV apex (Klues, Schiffers, and Maron 1995). Although HCM is typically characterized by asymmetric septal hypertrophy (ASH), almost any myocardial segment may be involved. Accurate assessment of LV wall thickness can be challenging when hypertrophy is confined to one or two segments, particularly in the anterolateral wall or the LV apex (Klues, Schiffers, and Maron 1995). Assessing the extent and severity of hypertrophy must include the measurement of maximal wall thickness in all LV segments from base to apex, ensuring that the wall thickness is recorded at mitral, mid-LV and apical levels. Localization of hypertrophy was established in accordance with the Maron's classification as follows (B. J. Maron, Gottdiener, and Epstein 1981): Type I pattern involving only the anteroseptum, Type II involving the whole septum wall, Type III involving the septum and, at least in part, the LV free wall, and Type IV involving other localizations (posterior, apex, or lateral wall). The following two-dimensional (2D) echocardiographic criteria are used to confirm diagnosis:

1. Unexplained maximal wall thickness ≥15 mm in any myocardial segment (Figure 2), or
2. Septal/posterior wall thickness ratio >1.3 in normotensive patients.

Nevertheless, genotype positive adults (including those who die suddenly) may have normal or near normal wall thickness.

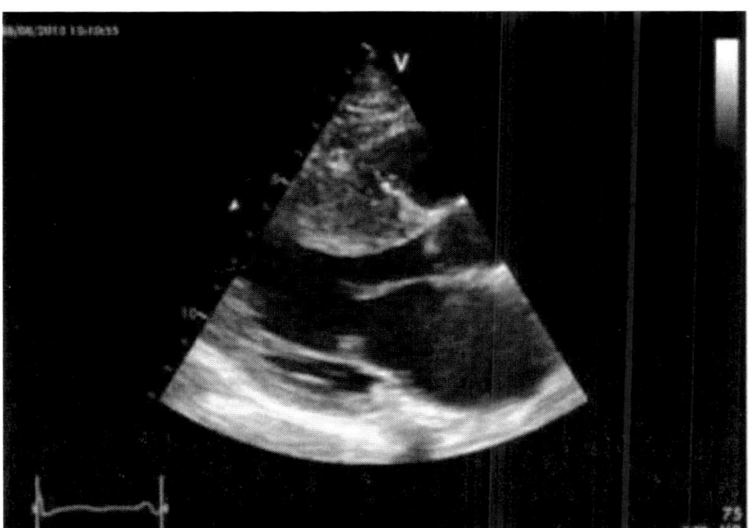

Figure 2. Parasternal long-axis view showing severe asymmetric septal hypertrophy.

However, it is important to recognize that asymmetric left ventricular hypertrophy (LVH) in itself is not pathognomonic of HCM but may be encountered in a variety of congenital or acquired conditions, including right ventricular hypertension, systemic hypertension, aortic stenosis, septal sarcomas, Fabry disease, Freidreich's ataxia, mucopolysaccharide or glycogen storage disorders and amyloidosis (Elliott et al. 2014).

Associated Abnormalities of Left Ventricular Outflow Tract

The pathophysiology of HCM is complex and consists of multiple interrelated abnormalities, including LVOT obstruction, diastolic dysfunction, mitral regurgitation, myocardial ischemia, and arrhythmias (Almenar et al. 1996). It is clinically important to distinguish between the obstructive and non-obstructive forms of HCM because management strategies are largely dependent on the presence or absence of symptoms caused by obstruction. For HCM, it is the peak instantaneous LV outflow gradient rather than the mean gradient that influences treatment decisions (Figure 3). Up to one third of patients with HCM will have obstruction under basal (resting) conditions (defined as gradients ≥30 mm Hg). Another one third will have labile, physiologically provoked gradients (<30 mm Hg at rest and ≥30 mm Hg with physiologic provocation) (Cotrim et al. 2011). The final one third will have the non-obstructive form of HCM (gradients <30 mm Hg at rest and with provocation). Marked gradients ≥50 mm Hg, either at rest or with provocation, represent the conventional threshold for surgical or percutaneous intervention if symptoms cannot be controlled with medication. The presence of SAM is documented using M-mode echocardiography and is characterized by mid-systolic notching of the aortic valve and contact of the anterior mitral valve leaflet/chordae with the septum (Figure 4).

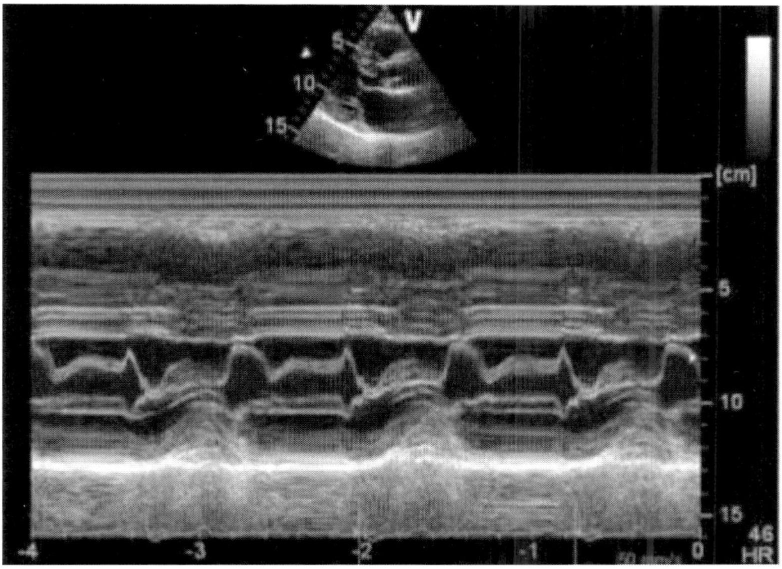

Figure 3. M-mode across the mitral leaflets showing the presence of systolic anterior motion of the anterior mitral leaflets (SAM).

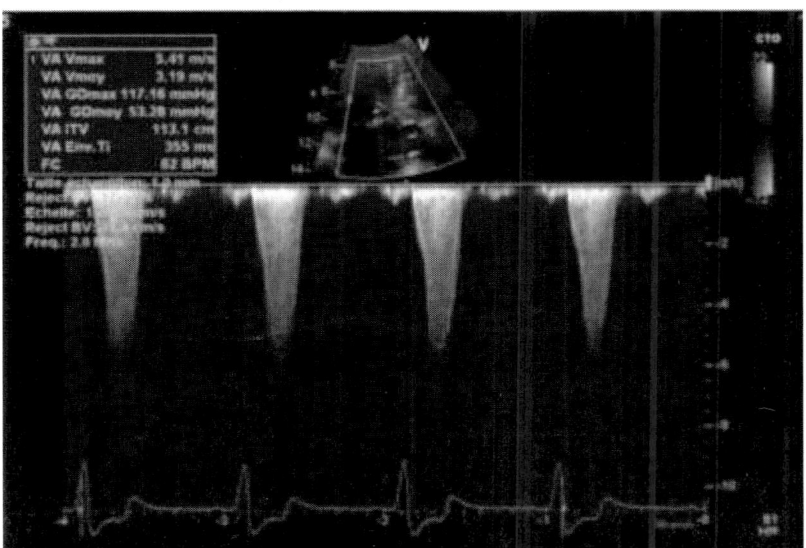

Figure 4. Late-peaking left ventricular outflow tract obstruction.

In obstructive HCM, the interventricular septum is much wider, with a smaller LV cavity, and greater incidence of mitral insufficiency, generally directed towards the posterior wall of the left atrium, and a larger tendency to calcify the mitral annulus. Obstruction to LV outflow is dynamic, varying with loading conditions and contractility of the ventricle. Increased myocardial contractility, decreased ventricular volume, or decreased afterload increase the degree of sub-aortic obstruction. Most recent studies that explain the mechanism of the outflow tract gradient in HCM emphasize that during ventricular systole, flow against the abnormally positioned mitral valve apparatus results in drag force on a portion of the mitral valve leaflets, which pushes the leaflets into the outflow tract. When a gradient is detected in the LV cavity, it is important to systematically exclude obstruction that is unrelated to SAM, including sub-aortic membranes, mitral valve leaflet abnormalities and mid-cavity obstruction, particularly when interventions to relieve LV outflow obstruction are contemplated.

Assessment of Latent Obstruction

Identification of LVOTO is important in the management of symptoms and assessment of sudden cardiac death risk. 2D and Doppler echocardiography during a Valsalva manoeuvre in the sitting and semi-supine position—and then on standing, if no gradient is provoked—is recommended for all patients (Minami et al. 2011). Exercise stress echocardiography is recommended in symptomatic patients if bedside manoeuvres fail to induce LVOTO ≥50 mm Hg. Pharmacological provocation with Dobutamine is not recommended, as it is not physiological and can be poorly tolerated. Similarly, nitrates do not reproduce exercise induced gradients and should be reserved for patients who cannot perform physiologically stressful procedures (Musat and Sherrid 2006). Mid-systolic notching, systolic fluttering of the aortic valve, and fibrotic septal changes at the level of leaflet-septal contact are related echocardiographic features in obstructive HCM.

Mitral Regurgitation

Systolic anterior motion of the mitral valve nearly always results in failure of normal leaflet coaptation and mitral regurgitation, which is typically mid-to-late systolic and inferolaterally oriented. The presence of a centrally or anteriorly directed jet of mitral regurgitation should raise suspicion of an intrinsic mitral valve abnormality and prompt further assessment with transoesophageal echocardiography, if necessary.

Left Atrial Enlargement

Left atrial (LA) volume is largely determined by the presence of diastolic dysfunction, mitral regurgitation, and atrial myopathy.

LA volume has been found to be a long-term independent indicator of functional capacity and an LA volume index of >34 ml/m^2 has been shown to be predictive of a greater degree of LVH, severity of diastolic dysfunction, and adverse cardiovascular outcomes.

Conventional Assessment of LV Systolic and Diastolic Functions

Left ventricular ejection fraction is usually preserved despite significant impairment of longitudinal contractile function, evidenced by attenuation in systolic annular velocities, strain and strain rate. Strain imaging can identify regional heterogeneity in contractile function, and clarify myocardial mechanics in HCM (Urbano-Moral et al. 2014). Terminally in the disease process, myocardial fibrosis may result in progressive impairment of systolic function end-stage HCM. Deterioration of systolic function has also been associated with increased mortality (up to 11% per year) and sudden cardiac death. A thorough assessment of systolic function by means of a biplane Simpson's ejection fraction and tissue Doppler imaging (TDI)-derived systolic velocities should be performed in the basal inferoseptal and anterolateral walls routinely in all patients at initial diagnosis and on subsequent scans. In patients with HCM, systolic function is typically normal or supernormal regardless of the presence of LVOT obstruction.

On the other hand, patients with HCM often have diastolic dysfunction, mostly indicating impaired myocardial relaxation regardless of symptoms or presence of LV outflow obstruction. Assessment of LV filling pressures is helpful in the evaluation of symptoms and disease staging. Doppler echocardiographic parameters are sensitive measures of diastolic function, but are influenced by loading conditions, heart rate and age. Therefore, a comprehensive evaluation of diastolic function, including Doppler of mitral valve inflow (E), tissue Doppler velocities at the mitral annulus (e'), pulmonary vein flow velocities, pulmonary artery systolic pressure and LA size and volume is recommended as part of the routine assessment of HCM. Variables recommended for evaluation of diastolic function in patients with HCM are average E/e' ratio (>14), LA volume index (>34 mL/m2), pulmonary vein atrial reversal velocity (Ar-A duration ≥30 msec), and peak velocity of tricuspid regurgitation (TR) jet by continuous-wave Doppler (>2.8 m/sec). The parameters can be applied irrespective of the presence or absence of dynamic obstruction and mitral regurgitation (MR), except for patients with more than moderate MR, in whom only Ar-A duration and peak velocity of TR jet are still valid (Nagueh et al. 2016).

Patients with a restrictive LV filling pattern may be at higher risk for adverse outcome, even with a preserved ejection fraction (EF).

Tissue Doppler Imaging (TDI)

TDI has become standard in most tertiary centres managing patients with cardiomyopathies. Systolic velocities are attenuated in HCM despite a preserved or supranormal ejection fraction, even in myocardial segments which do not demonstrate overt hypertrophy. The early-diastolic mitral annular velocity (e') is reduced in HCM patients with the degree of attenuation related to the magnitude of hypertrophy. TDI may also help in differentiating various conditions resulting in LVH, with demonstrable differences in TDI velocities between conditions of physiological hypertrophy (athlete's heart) and pathological hypertrophy. Mean systolic annular motion S'<9 cm/s is a parameter for differentiating pathological LVH (HCM/hypertensive LVH) from physiological LVH (diagnostic accuracy of 92%). In a recent report of patients with established HCM, low lateral mitral annular systolic velocity (<4 cm/s) was found to have prognostic value and independently predicted death or hospitalization for worsening heart failure (Vinereanu et al. 2001). However, tissue Doppler imaging is an angle-dependent technique, influenced by cardiac translational motion and tethering. The evolution of newer echocardiographic technologies such as strain imaging, speckle tracking, and 3D echocardiography (3D-E) has revolutionized the assessment of cardiac performance from assessment of ejection fraction to a more sophisticated assessment of regional cardiac mechanics. These advances have facilitated preclinical diagnosis, improved risk stratification and contributed to our understanding of therapeutic options for HCM.

2D Strain or Speckle Tracking Imaging

2D strain allows spatial and temporal tracking of longitudinal, circumferential and radial myocardial deformation. Its ability to provide angle-independent measures of LV strain is advantageous. Studies in patients with HCM have demonstrated a reduction in longitudinal strain with basal to apical gradient (Figure 5), an increase in circumferential strain, normal systolic twist or torsion, and reduction in untwisting in diastole. Significant reductions in strain in the LV septal segments (particularly the mid-septal segment) correlate with the septal/posterior wall ratio (Serri et al. 2006). Longitudinal deformation abnormalities are often focal or sub-segmental and may be underestimated if careful spatial mapping is not used. Because of its intrinsic ability to provide angle-independent strain data, 2D strain holds a unique advantage over tissue Doppler-derived strain, which is particularly important for myocardial deformation analysis in the apical LV segments.

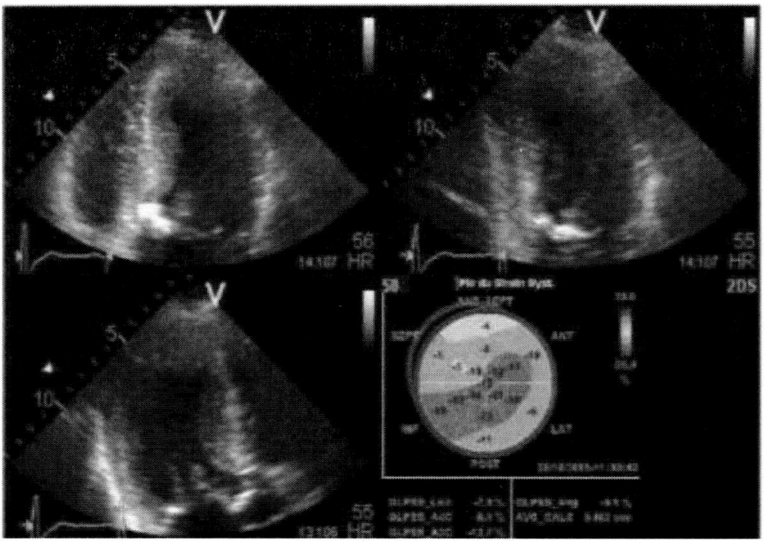

Figure 5. Two-dimensional strain images showing paradoxical apical longitudinal strain and corresponding abnormalities in the color M-mode of the parametric strain map. Loss of base-apex (strain) gradient is present.

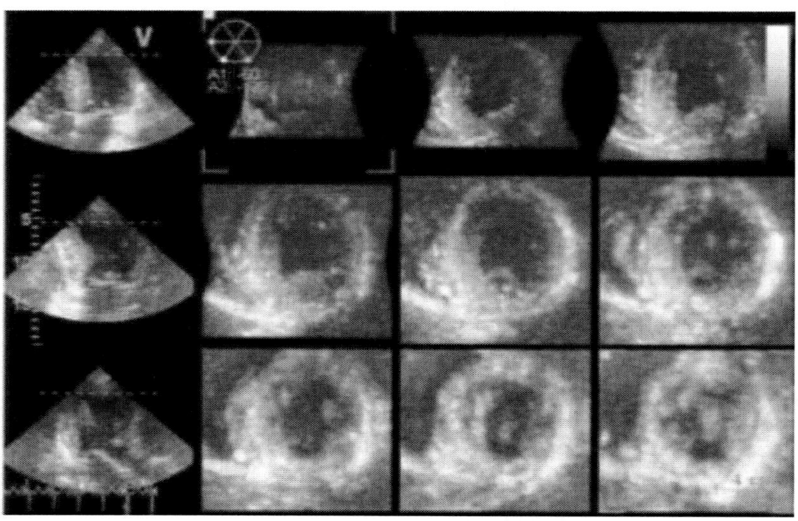

Figure 6. Three-dimensional echocardiography showing asymmetric left ventricle hypertrophy.

Three-Dimensional Echocardiography

3D-echocardiography (Figure 6) has provided insights into the mechanics of SAM and deformational geometry of the LV outflow tract. This method facilitates the assessment of the LVOT area after intervention for septal reduction, surgical myectomy, volumetric estimates of left atrial mechanical function, and accurate estimation of LV ejection fraction as well as LV mass in hypertrophied hearts (comparing favourably with CMR imaging).

Trans-Oesophageal Echocardiography

Trans-oesophageal echocardiography (TEE) should be considered in patients with poor transthoracic echo windows, as an alternative or complementary investigation to CMR. It is particularly useful in patients with LVOTO if the mechanism is unclear, when assessing the mitral valve apparatus before a septal reduction procedure, and when severe mitral regurgitation caused by intrinsic valve abnormalities is suspected. In patients undergoing septal myectomy, perioperative TEE should be used to guide the surgical strategy and to detect surgical complications (ventricular septal defect and aortic regurgitation (AR) and residual LVOTO. Following myectomy, intraoperative TEE studies can confirm the adequacy of myectomy and quantitate residual gradients, severity of mitral and aortic regurgitation, ventricular function, and development of a ventricular septal defect (Soor et al. 2009).

Contrast Echocardiography

Contrast echocardiography is currently used to enhance endocardial definition, Doppler signals, and to evaluate myocardial perfusion. Myocardial contrast echocardiography can help anticipate the location and delineate the extent of septal infarct (selective injection of contrast into septal perforators) before alcohol septal ablation.

Differential Diagnosis

Differential diagnosis between HCM and physiologic non-pathologic left ventricular (LV) hypertrophy associated with physical training (commonly referred to as "athlete's heart") has important implications, because identification of cardiovascular diseases associated with sudden death may be the basis for disqualification from competition to minimize risk. Conversely, improper over-diagnosis of cardiac disease may lead to unnecessary withdrawal from athletics. Echocardiography is one of the most important methods for differentiation between pathologic and physiologic left ventricular hypertrophy (B. J. Maron 2009).

Echocardiographic criteria favouring HCM:

- Systolic mitral annual velocity <9cm/sec
- Diastolic dysfunction
- Lack of LVH regression after cessation of exercise
- Lack of LV dilatation
- Provocable LVOT gradient
- Attenuated longitudinal, circumferential and radial strains (2D Strain)
- Intraventricular dyssynchrony

Common diagnostic challenges in echocardiography include the following:

- Presentation in the late phase of the disease with a dilated and/or hypokinetic left ventricle and LV wall thinning
- Physiological hypertrophy caused by intense athletic training
- Patients with co-existent pathologies
- Isolated basal septal hypertrophy in elderly people

In conclusion, conventional echocardiography (TTE) is the most readily accessible and informative tool in making a diagnosis of HCM. It is also the first non-invasive imaging method for risk stratification, treatment, selection and follow-up of the patients. Two-dimensional strain is a simple, rapid, and reproducible method of early detection of abnormalities in patients with HCM that have apparently normal left ventricular systolic function.

Cardiovascular Magnetic Resonance Imaging

Cardiovascular magnetic resonance (CMR) imaging embraces several modalities that provide detailed information on cardiac morphology, ventricular function and myocardial tissue characteristics (O'Hanlon, Assomull, and Prasad 2007).

Assessment of Ventricular Morphology and Function

In patients with good echocardiographic images, CMR provides similar information on ventricular function and morphology (Olivotto et al. 2008), but it can be helpful in establishing the diagnosis of HCM in patients with poor acoustic windows or when some LV regions are poorly visualized—such as the anterolateral wall, the LV apex and the right ventricle (Rickers et al. 2005). As in 2D echocardiography, over-estimation of wall thickness can result from oblique sections (particularly at the LV apex) or from inclusion of paraseptal structures such as the moderator band or false tendons. Over-estimation of wall thickness is also possible in spoiled gradient echo images and so, steady-state free precession (SSFP) cine sequences are preferred. Cardiovascular magnetic resonance imaging is superior to transthoracic echocardiography (TTE) in the measurement of LV mass, but LV mass itself correlates weakly with maximal wall thickness and can be normal in patients with asymmetric HCM, especially when it involves less than two LV segments (Spiewak et al. 2010).

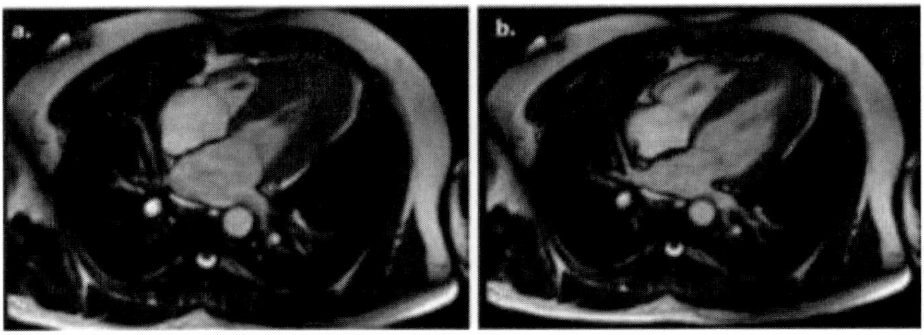

Figure 7. (a and b). Cardiovascular magnetic resonance imaging showing left ventricle apical hypertrophy.

CMR imaging is superior to standard 2D echocardiography in the detection of LV apical and anterolateral hypertrophy (Figure 7), aneurysms (M. S. Maron et al. 2008) and thrombi (Weinsaft et al. 2011) and is more sensitive in the detection of subtle markers of disease, such as myocardial crypts and papillary muscle abnormalities in patients with sarcomeric protein gene mutations (Brouwer et al. 2012). Phase velocity flow mapping sequences can be used to determine the peak velocity of blood flow through the LV outflow tract in patients with LVOTO, but proper alignment of the imaging plane to obtain the highest flow velocities is time-consuming and prone to error. For these reasons, Doppler echocardiography is the modality of choice for quantification of LVOTO. Similarly, while mitral inflow velocities and pulmonary vein flow derived from phase contrast CMR (PC-CMR) provide highly reproducible and accurate data in experienced hands, echocardiography is the preferred method for assessment of diastolic function in routine practice (Nagueh et al. 2016). CMR can quantify the amount of tissue necrosis induced by septal alcohol ablation, as well as the location of scarring and the regression of LV mass following the procedure (Valeti et al. 2007).

Myocardial Fibrosis

By using the intrinsic magnetic properties of different tissues and the distribution of gadolinium-based contrast agents, CMR can be used to detect expansion of the myocardial interstitium caused by fibrosis. Late gadolinium enhancement is unusual in non-hypertrophied segments except in advanced stages of the disease, when full-thickness LGE in association with wall thinning is common (Valeti et al. 2007). Late gadolinium enhancement may be associated with increased myocardial stiffness and adverse LV remodelling, and the extent of LGE is associated with a higher incidence of regional wall motion abnormalities.

On balance, the extent of LGE on CMR has some utility in predicting cardiovascular mortality, but current data do not support the use of LGE to predict SCD risk (Elliott et al. 2014).

Differential Diagnosis

Cardiac magnetic resonance imaging rarely distinguishes the causes of HCM by their magnetic properties alone, but the distribution and severity of interstitial expansion can, in context, suggest specific diagnoses.

The absence of fibrosis may be helpful in differentiating HCM from physiological adaptation in athletes, but LGE may be absent in people with HCM, particularly the young and those with mild disease (Elliott et al. 2014).

Cardiac Computerized Tomography

The high contrast resolution of computerized tomography (CT) provides clear imaging of the myocardium and accurate measurement of wall thickness, ventricular volumes, ejection fraction and LV mass, which correlate well with CMR and echocardiography (Schroeder et al. 2008). Cardiovascular CT permits the simultaneous imaging of the coronary arteries and valves (Schroeder et al. 2008). Cardiac CT should be considered in patients for whom there are inadequate echocardiographic imaging and contraindications for CMR (Elliott et al. 2014).

Laboratory Tests

Routine laboratory testing aids the detection of extra-cardiac conditions that cause or exacerbate ventricular dysfunction (for example, thyroid disease, renal dysfunction and diabetes mellitus) and secondary organ dysfunction in patients with severe heart failure. High levels of brain natriuretic peptide (BNP) (Geske et al. 2013), N-terminal pro-brain natriuretic peptide (NT-proBNP) (Coats et al. 2013) and high sensitivity cardiac troponin T (hs-cTnT) are associated with cardiovascular events, heart failure and death. Despite comparable values of ventricular wall thickness, plasma BNP values are three to five times as high in patients with cardiac amyloidosis as those in other causes of HCM.

Genetic Testing

In the majority of cases, HCM is inherited as an autosomal dominant genetic trait with a 50% risk of transmission to offspring (Richard et al. 2003).

Genetic testing, which is now commercially available, is a powerful strategy for definitive diagnosis of affected genetic status and is currently used most effectively in the identification of affected relatives in families known to have HCM (Elliott et al. 2014).

Conclusion

Hypertrophic cardiomyopathy (HCM) is a genetic disorder that is characterized by commonly asymmetrical left ventricular hypertrophy (LVH). HCM is an important cause of sudden cardiac death, particularly in adolescents and young adults. Most patients with HCM are asymptomatic but some develop symptoms, often many years after the appearance of electrocardiographic or echocardiographic evidence of LVH.

The diagnosis of HCM is most often established with any noninvasive cardiac imaging modality, especially transthoracic echocardiography and/or cardiac magnetic resonance imaging.

REFERENCES

Adabag, A. Selcuk, Susan A. Casey, Michael A. Kuskowski, Andrey G. Zenovich, and Barry J. Maron. 2005. "Spectrum and Prognostic Significance of Arrhythmias on Ambulatory Holter Electrocardiogram in Hypertrophic Cardiomyopathy." *Journal of the American College of Cardiology* 45 (5): 697–704. doi:10.1016/j.jacc.2004.11.043.

Almenar, L., S. Martí, I. Roldán, V. Miró, J. L. Díez, A. Osa, M. Palencia, and F. Algarra. 1996. "(Obstructive and non-obstructive hypertrophic cardiomyopathy: clinical, electrocardiographic, and echocardiographic differences)." *Revista Espanola De Cardiologia* 49 (6): 423–31.

Authors/Task Force members, Perry M. Elliott, Aris Anastasakis, Michael A. Borger, Martin Borggrefe, Franco Cecchi, Philippe Charron, et al. 2014. "2014 ESC Guidelines on Diagnosis and Management of Hypertrophic Cardiomyopathy: The Task Force for the Diagnosis and Management of Hypertrophic Cardiomyopathy of the European Society of Cardiology (ESC)." *European Heart Journal* 35 (39): 2733–79. doi:10.1093/eurheartj/ehu284.

Brouwer, Wessel P., Tjeerd Germans, Maaike C. Head, Jolanda van der Velden, Martijn W. Heymans, Imke Christiaans, Arjan C. Houweling, Arthur A. Wilde, and Albert C. van Rossum. 2012. "Multiple Myocardial Crypts on Modified Long-Axis View Are a Specific Finding in Pre-Hypertrophic HCM Mutation Carriers." *European Heart Journal Cardiovascular Imaging* 13 (4): 292–97. doi:10.1093/ehjci/jes005.

Charron, P., J. F. Forissier, M. E. Amara, O. Dubourg, M. Desnos, J. B. Bouhour, R. Isnard, et al. 2003. "Accuracy of European Diagnostic Criteria for Familial Hypertrophic Cardiomyopathy in a Genotyped

Population." *International Journal of Cardiology* 90 (1): 33–38; discussion 38–40.

Coats, Caroline J., Mathew J. Gallagher, Michael Foley, Constantinos O'Mahony, Christopher Critoph, Juan Gimeno, Anne Dawnay, William J. McKenna, and Perry M. Elliott. 2013. "Relation between Serum N-Terminal pro-Brain Natriuretic Peptide and Prognosis in Patients with Hypertrophic Cardiomyopathy." *European Heart Journal* 34 (32): 2529–37. doi:10.1093/eurheartj/eht070.

Cotrim, Carlos, Ana Rita Almeida, Luís Lopes, Paula Fazendas, Isabel João, and Hélder Pereira. 2011. "What Is Really a Nonobstructive Hypertrophic Cardiomyopathy? The Importance of Orthostatic Factor in Exercise Echocardiography." *ISRN Cardiology* 2011: 346797. doi:10.5402/2011/346797.

Feiner, Ellina, Milla Arabadjian, Glenda Winson, Bette Kim, Farooq Chaudhry, and Mark V. Sherrid. 2013. "Post-Prandial Upright Exercise Echocardiography in Hypertrophic Cardiomyopathy." *Journal of the American College of Cardiology* 61 (24): 2487–88. doi:10.1016/j.jacc.2013.02.079.

Gersh, Bernard J., Barry J. Maron, Robert O. Bonow, Joseph A. Dearani, Michael A. Fifer, Mark S. Link, Srihari S. Naidu, et al. 2011. "2011 ACCF/AHA Guideline for the Diagnosis and Treatment of Hypertrophic Cardiomyopathy: A Report of the American College of Cardiology Foundation/American Heart Association Task Force on Practice Guidelines. Developed in Collaboration with the American Association for Thoracic Surgery, American Society of Echocardiography, American Society of Nuclear Cardiology, Heart Failure Society of America, Heart Rhythm Society, Society for Cardiovascular Angiography and Interventions, and Society of Thoracic Surgeons." *Journal of the American College of Cardiology* 58 (25): e212–60. doi:10.1016/j.jacc.2011.06.011.

Geske, Jeffrey B., Paul M. McKie, Steve R. Ommen, and Paul Sorajja. 2013. "B-Type Natriuretic Peptide and Survival in Hypertrophic Cardiomyopathy." *Journal of the American College of Cardiology* 61 (24): 2456–60. doi:10.1016/j.jacc.2013.04.004.

Gilligan, D. M., P. Nihoyannopoulos, A. Fletcher, E. Sbarouni, A. Dritsas, and C. M. Oakley. 1996. "Symptoms of Hypertrophic Cardiomyopathy, with Special Emphasis on Syncope and Postprandial Exacerbation of Symptoms." *Clinical Cardiology* 19 (5): 371–78.

Gimeno, Juan R., Maite Tomé-Esteban, Carla Lofiego, José Hurtado, Antonios Pantazis, Bryan Mist, Pier Lambiase, William J. McKenna, and Perry M. Elliott. 2009. "Exercise-Induced Ventricular Arrhythmias and Risk of Sudden Cardiac Death in Patients with Hypertrophic Cardiomyopathy." *European Heart Journal* 30 (21): 2599–2605. doi:10.1093/eurheartj/ehp327.

Klues, H. G., A. Schiffers, and B. J. Maron. 1995. "Phenotypic Spectrum and Patterns of Left Ventricular Hypertrophy in Hypertrophic Cardiomyopathy: Morphologic Observations and Significance as Assessed by Two-Dimensional Echocardiography in 600 Patients." *Journal of the American College of Cardiology* 26 (7): 1699–1708. doi:10.1016/0735-1097(95)00390-8.

Maron, B. J. 2009. "Distinguishing Hypertrophic Cardiomyopathy from Athlete's Heart Physiological Remodelling: Clinical Significance, Diagnostic Strategies and Implications for Preparticipation Screening." *British Journal of Sports Medicine* 43 (9): 649–56. doi: 10.1136/bjsm.2008.054726.

Maron, B. J., J. S. Gottdiener, and S. E. Epstein. 1981. "Patterns and Significance of Distribution of Left Ventricular Hypertrophy in Hypertrophic Cardiomyopathy. A Wide Angle, Two Dimensional Echocardiographic Study of 125 Patients." *The American Journal of Cardiology* 48 (3): 418–28.

Maron, Martin S., John J. Finley, J. Martijn Bos, Thomas H. Hauser, Warren J. Manning, Tammy S. Haas, John R. Lesser, James E. Udelson, Michael J. Ackerman, and Barry J. Maron. 2008. "Prevalence, Clinical Significance, and Natural History of Left Ventricular Apical Aneurysms in Hypertrophic Cardiomyopathy." *Circulation* 118 (15): 1541–49. doi:10.1161/CIRCULATIONAHA. 108.781401.

McLeod, Christopher J., Michael J. Ackerman, Rick A. Nishimura, A. Jamil Tajik, Bernard J. Gersh, and Steve R. Ommen. 2009. "Outcome of Patients with Hypertrophic Cardiomyopathy and a Normal Electrocardiogram." *Journal of the American College of Cardiology* 54 (3): 229–33. doi:10.1016/j.jacc.2009.02.071.

Minami, Yuichiro, Katsuya Kajimoto, Yutaka Terajima, Bun Yashiro, Dai Okayama, Shintaro Haruki, Takatomo Nakajima, Naomi Kawashiro, Masatoshi Kawana, and Nobuhisa Hagiwara. 2011. "Clinical Implications of Midventricular Obstruction in Patients with Hypertrophic Cardiomyopathy." *Journal of the American College of Cardiology* 57 (23): 2346–55. doi:10.1016/j.jacc.2011.02.033.

Monserrat, Lorenzo, Perry M. Elliott, Juan R. Gimeno, Sanjay Sharma, Manuel Penas-Lado, and William J. McKenna. 2003. "Non-Sustained Ventricular Tachycardia in Hypertrophic Cardiomyopathy: An Independent Marker of Sudden Death Risk in Young Patients." *Journal of the American College of Cardiology* 42 (5): 873–79.

Musat, Dan, and Mark V. Sherrid. 2006. "Echocardiography in the Treatment of Hypertrophic Cardiomyopathy." *Anadolu Kardiyoloji Dergisi: AKD = the Anatolian Journal of Cardiology* 6 Suppl 2 (December): 18–26.

Nagueh, Sherif F., Otto A. Smiseth, Christopher P. Appleton, Benjamin F. Byrd, Hisham Dokainish, Thor Edvardsen, Frank A. Flachskampf, et al. 2016. "Recommendations for the Evaluation of Left Ventricular Diastolic Function by Echocardiography: An Update from the American Society of Echocardiography and the European Association of Cardiovascular Imaging." *Journal of the American Society of Echocardiography: Official Publication of the American Society of Echocardiography* 29 (4): 277–314. doi:10.1016/j.echo.2016.01.011.

O'Hanlon, Rory, Ravi G. Assomull, and Sanjay K. Prasad. 2007. "Use of Cardiovascular Magnetic Resonance for Diagnosis and Management in Hypertrophic Cardiomyopathy." *Current Cardiology Reports* 9 (1): 51–56.

Olivotto, Iacopo, Martin S. Maron, Camillo Autore, John R. Lesser, Luigi Rega, Giancarlo Casolo, Marcello De Santis, et al. 2008. "Assessment and Significance of Left Ventricular Mass by Cardiovascular Magnetic Resonance in Hypertrophic Cardiomyopathy." *Journal of the American College of Cardiology* 52 (7): 559–66. doi: 10.1016/j.jacc.2008.04.047.

Paz, R., R. Jortner, P. A. Tunick, S. Sclarovsky, B. Eilat, J. L. Perez, and I. Kronzon. 1996. "The Effect of the Ingestion of Ethanol on Obstruction of the Left Ventricular Outflow Tract in Hypertrophic Cardiomyopathy." *The New England Journal of Medicine* 335 (13): 938–41. doi:10.1056/NEJM199609263351305.

Richard, Pascale, Philippe Charron, Lucie Carrier, Céline Ledeuil, Theary Cheav, Claire Pichereau, Abdelaziz Benaiche, et al. 2003. "Hypertrophic Cardiomyopathy: Distribution of Disease Genes, Spectrum of Mutations, and Implications for a Molecular Diagnosis Strategy." *Circulation* 107 (17): 2227–32. doi:10.1161/01.CIR. 0000066323.15244.54.

Rickers, Carsten, Norbert M. Wilke, Michael Jerosch-Herold, Susan A. Casey, Prasad Panse, Neeta Panse, Jochen Weil, Andrey G. Zenovich, and Barry J. Maron. 2005. "Utility of Cardiac Magnetic Resonance Imaging in the Diagnosis of Hypertrophic Cardiomyopathy." *Circulation* 112 (6): 855–61. doi:10.1161/CIRCULATIONAHA. 104.507723.

Schroeder, Stephen, Stephan Achenbach, Frank Bengel, Christof Burgstahler, Filippo Cademartiri, Pim de Feyter, Richard George, et al. 2008. "Cardiac Computed Tomography: Indications, Applications, Limitations, and Training Requirements: Report of a Writing Group Deployed by the Working Group Nuclear Cardiology and Cardiac CT of the European Society of Cardiology and the European Council of Nuclear Cardiology." *European Heart Journal* 29 (4): 531–56. doi:10.1093/eurheartj/ehm544.

Serri, Karim, Patricia Reant, Marianne Lafitte, Marianne Berhouet, Valerie Le Bouffos, Raymond Roudaut, and Stephane Lafitte. 2006. "Global and Regional Myocardial Function Quantification by Two-Dimensional Strain: Application in Hypertrophic Cardiomyopathy."

Journal of the American College of Cardiology 47 (6): 1175–81. doi:10.1016/j.jacc.2005.10.061.

Shah, J. S., M. T. T. Esteban, R. Thaman, R. Sharma, B. Mist, A. Pantazis, D. Ward, et al. 2008. "Prevalence of Exercise-Induced Left Ventricular Outflow Tract Obstruction in Symptomatic Patients with Non-Obstructive Hypertrophic Cardiomyopathy." *Heart (British Cardiac Society)* 94 (10): 1288–94. doi:10.1136/hrt.2007.126003.

Soor, G. S., A. Luk, E. Ahn, J. R. Abraham, A. Woo, A. Ralph-Edwards, and J. Butany. 2009. "Hypertrophic Cardiomyopathy: Current Understanding and Treatment Objectives." *Journal of Clinical Pathology* 62 (3): 226–35. doi:10.1136/jcp.2008.061655.

Sorajja, Paul, Steve R. Ommen, Rick A. Nishimura, Bernard J. Gersh, Peter B. Berger, and A. Jamil Tajik. 2003. "Adverse Prognosis of Patients with Hypertrophic Cardiomyopathy Who Have Epicardial Coronary Artery Disease." *Circulation* 108 (19): 2342–48. doi:10.1161/01.CIR.0000097110.55312.BF.

Spiewak, Mateusz, Lidia Chojnowska, Lukasz A. Małek, Barbara Miłosz, Joanna Petryka, Magdalena Zabicka, Mariusz Kłopotowski, Maciej Dabrowski, Jolanta Miśko, and Witold Ruzyłło. 2010. "Comparison between Maximal Left Ventricular Wall Thickness and Left Ventricular Mass in Patients with Hypertrophic Cardiomyopathy." *Kardiologia Polska* 68 (7): 763–68.

Task Force for the Diagnosis and Management of Syncope, European Society of Cardiology (ESC), European Heart Rhythm Association (EHRA), Heart Failure Association (HFA), Heart Rhythm Society (HRS), Angel Moya, Richard Sutton, et al. 2009. "Guidelines for the Diagnosis and Management of Syncope (version 2009)." *European Heart Journal* 30 (21): 2631–71. doi:10.1093/eurheartj/ehp298.

Urbano-Moral, Jose Angel, Ethan J. Rowin, Martin S. Maron, Andrew Crean, and Natesa G. Pandian. 2014. "Investigation of Global and Regional Myocardial Mechanics with 3-Dimensional Speckle Tracking Echocardiography and Relations to Hypertrophy and Fibrosis in Hypertrophic Cardiomyopathy." *Circulation. Cardiovascular Imaging* 7 (1): 11–19. doi:10.1161/CIRCIMAGING.113.000842.

Valeti, Uma S., Rick A. Nishimura, David R. Holmes, Philip A. Araoz, James F. Glockner, Jerome F. Breen, Steve R. Ommen, et al. 2007. "Comparison of Surgical Septal Myectomy and Alcohol Septal Ablation with Cardiac Magnetic Resonance Imaging in Patients with Hypertrophic Obstructive Cardiomyopathy." *Journal of the American College of Cardiology* 49 (3): 350–57. doi:10.1016/j.jacc.2006.08.055.

Vinereanu, D., N. Florescu, N. Sculthorpe, A. C. Tweddel, M. R. Stephens, and A. G. Fraser. 2001. "Differentiation between Pathologic and Physiologic Left Ventricular Hypertrophy by Tissue Doppler Assessment of Long-Axis Function in Patients with Hypertrophic Cardiomyopathy or Systemic Hypertension and in Athletes." *The American Journal of Cardiology* 88 (1): 53–58.

Weinsaft, Jonathan W., Han W. Kim, Anna Lisa Crowley, Igor Klem, Chetan Shenoy, Lowie Van Assche, Rhoda Brosnan, et al. 2011. "LV Thrombus Detection by Routine Echocardiography: Insights into Performance Characteristics Using Delayed Enhancement CMR." *JACC. Cardiovascular Imaging* 4 (7): 702–12. doi:10.1016/j.jcmg.2011.03.017.

In: Hypertrophic Cardiomyopathy
Editor: Ikram Kammoun
ISBN: 978-1-53613-003-4

Chapter 3

Atrial Fibrillation in Hypertrophic Cardiomyopathy

Françoise Hidden-Lucet[1,*], MD and Estelle Gandjbakhch[2], MD, PhD

[1]Department of Cardiology, ICAN University Hospital Institute, APHP, Paris, France

[2]Department of Cardiology, Pierre and Marie CURIE – University PARIS VI, ICAN University Hospital Institute, APHP, Paris, France

Abstract

Atrial fibrillation (AF) is the most common disease complication of hypertrophic cardiomyopathy, occurring 4- to 6- fold more often than in the general population and at a younger age. Major determinants for AF occurrence are age, and LA size and function. AF is frequently poorly tolerated and is an independent predictor of overall mortality, mainly due to stroke and heart failure. Therefore, lifelong antithrombotic therapy is recommended after a first AF episode regardless of CHA_2DS_2VASc score. Repeated screening for AF occurrence with connected tools may be a valuable strategy for preventing embolic events in selected patients.

* Corresponding author: francoise.hidden-lucet@aphp.fr.

In symptomatic patients, restoring sinus rhythm is warranted but long-term antiarrhythmic therapy can be limited by poor efficacy, proarrhythmic risk, or toxicity in case of amiodarone. Although less efficient than in the general population, catheter ablation may be a valuable option for young patients with a short duration of AF and a mild LA dilatation. A stand-alone AF surgical procedure or a hybrid approach associated with left atrial appendage occlusion could benefit symptomatic patients with dilated atria and should be investigated.

Keywords: hypertrophic cardiomyopathy, atrial fibrillation, catheter ablation

INTRODUCTION

Hypertrophic cardiomyopathy (HCM) is a genetic disease characterised by the presence of a left ventricular hypertrophy in the absence of abnormal loading conditions. Preventing sudden cardiac death and managing left ventricular outflow tract (LVOT) obstruction have traditionally been the key priorities of HCM management. However, atrial fibrillation (AF) is much more common in HCM patients than ventricular arrhythmias and medically refractory obstruction, and is frequently poorly tolerated (Vaidya, Semsarian and Chan 2017). This chapter covers a range of issues concerning AF in patients with HCM, with a focus on prognosis, pathophysiology, and management.

PREVALENCE AND INCIDENCE

AF is the most common disease complication of HCM, occurring in 18 to 28% of patients which is 4- to 6- fold more common than in the general population (MacIntyre and Lakdawala 2016). In a retrospective study of 3,505 patients in sinus rhythm at baseline, 5- and 10- year cumulative incidence rates of AF were 16.0% (95%CI 14.6% to 17.5%) and 33.3% (95%CI 30.7% to 36.1%), respectively (Guttmann et al. 2017). Annual incidence is generally estimated around 2 to 3% and may be even greater in apical cardiomyopathy (Lee et al. 2017; Olivotto et al. 2001) and extensive septal hypertrophy (Park et al. 2016). AF onset is at age 55 on average, 10 years earlier than in the general population, one third of patients being diagnosed before the age of 50. More importantly, recent studies have emphasized the fact that silent AF occurs in 25% to 33% of patients implanted with an electronic device (Rowin et al. 2017; Wilke et al. 2016) with an annual incidence of 7% (van Velzen et al. 2017), thus posing a potential thromboembolic risk leading to disability or death.

PROGNOSIS

AF is associated with worse symptoms, lower exercise capacity, and is an independent predictor of overall mortality in HCM patients, increasing the risk of death four-fold compared to sinus rhythm (Vaidya, Semsarian, et Chan 2017; Siontis et al. 2014). In a recent retrospective longitudinal cohort of more than 4,000 patients, cardiovascular death reached 10.9% in AF patients compared to 4.9% in patients in sinus rhythm over a 10-year follow-up. Mortality rate was also higher in permanent and persistent AF than in paroxysmal AF (difference in proportion = 8.1%; 95%CI (4.5% to 11.7%)) (Guttmann et al. 2017). Younger age (<50 years) at AF occurrence is associated with a worse prognosis with a 1.7-fold related mortality, 3.6-fold related stroke prevalence and 1.5-fold progression of symptoms in 5 years of follow-up in comparison with late AF development (>50 years)

AF mortality is mainly driven by an increase in heart failure and stroke. Nevertheless, in a recent meta-analysis, Masri pointed out the fact that after excluding stroke-related deaths, AF was still associated with increased mortality, raising the question of association between sudden death and AF (Masri et al. 2017). However, no evidence is available yet to suggest that atrial fibrillation is an independant determinant of sudden death (Olivotto et al. 2001; Gersh et al. 2011). Stroke and ischemic embolic events are frequent in HCM, ischemic stroke being 8 times more frequent in patients with AF (21%) compared with those in sinus rhythm (2.6%). The prevalence of stroke is independant of whether the AF is paroxysmal or chronic (22% versus 27%) (Olivotto et al. 2001). As in the general population, AF-related strokes increase with age with an annual incidence rising from 0.8% to1.9% for patients ≥60 years old (Maron 2002).

Pathophysiology and AF Significance

Susceptibility to AF is merely linked to ageing and left-atrial enlargement. HCM patients are prone to adverse remodeling due to increased filling pressure secondary to LV diastolic dysfunction and hypertrophy as well as mitral regurgitation and LVOT obstruction (Debonnaire et al. 2017). Increased atrial fibrosis and atrial myofibril disarray favours AF (Vaidya, Semsarian, and Chan 2017). Specific sarcomeric mutations (Gruver et al. 1999) as well as polymorphism in the angiotensin-receptor gene have also been linked to the development of AF in patients with HCM (Tuluce and Tuluce 2015). In HCM patients with paroxysmal AF, exercise capacity in sinus rhythm is reduced compared with patients free of AF with equal left atrial volume (Azarbal et al. 2014; Owens 2014). It seems therefore likely that AF is an early marker of an intrinsic advanced disease, favouring disease progression over time.

Determinants of AF and AF Screening

Left atrial (LA) diameter, volume and function (as measured by LA strain) are all predictors of AF. For Olivotto, a LA diameter ≥45 mm is the threshold value associated with substantial risk of developing AF (Olivotto et al. 2001). The European Society of Cardiology recommends a 48-h ambulatory electrocardiogram monitoring every 6-12 months to detect AF in HCM patients who are in sinus rhythm and have a LA-diameter ≥45 mm. For Debonnaire, over 50% of HCM patients develop new-onset AF despite preserving a baseline LA diameter of <45 mm. Therefore, LA volume (≥37 ml/m2) and strain (≤23.4%), which improve prediction of new-onset AF, should be preferred over diameter for risk stratification (Debonnaire et al. 2017). A LA cutoff volume of >118 ml has also been reported to predict the occurrence of AF with 71% sensitivity and 65% specificity (Maron et al. 2014). LA functions and volumes should therefore be carefully monitored over time to identify individuals at risk before the onset of AF.

Heart failure symptoms and age are also strong predictors of AF development with an increased occurrence risk after 40 years old (Tuluce and Tuluce 2015). Confounding data has been reported in studies assessing the effect of LVOT obstruction on AF development, as well as myocardial fibrosis quantification and BNP levels. Therefore, these parameters are not routinely used in clinics to assess individual risk of AF occurrence in HCM patients. Finally, HCM has been reported to be associated with a high prevalence of obstructive sleep apnea that can favour AF (Eleid et al. 2009). Whether treating apnea would reduce AF burden in that population remains to be seen. As silent AF has been reported as much as 25 to 33% in HCM patients implanted with electronic devices, it is likely that asymptomatic AF is underestimated in device-free patients,thus leading to risk of stroke. In selected patients, close careful ECG monitoring using electronic devices and teletransmission might be useful for AF detection (Steinberg et al. 2017).

MANAGEMENT OF AF IN HCM

HCM patients are frequently more symptomatic of AF than the general population, and persistent AF may be responsible for acute heart failure decompensation, especially in case of rapid ventricular rate and LVOT obstruction. This warrants a more aggressive approach to restoration and maintenance of sinus rhythm (MacIntyre and Lakdawala 2016; Gersh et al. 2011; Tuluce and Tuluce 2015). Lifestyle changes and treatment aim to improve AF tolerance and limit AF burden. Risk factor management as well as dietary, weight loss and obstructive sleep apnea treatment should be undertaken as adjuvant therapy to limit AF recurrence. Furthermore, patients with HCM and AF are at higher risk of a thromboebolic event. The key points of AF management in those patients include thromboembolic prophylaxis as well as rate and rhythm control.

Anti-Thrombotic Treatment

Although not completely protective against systemic embolization, wafarin has been associated with a lower risk of stroke and is more efficacious than antiplatelet agents in HCM (Gruver et al. 1999; Guttmann et al. 2015). NOACs have not been compared to wafarin in these patients, but large observational datasets have shown a comparative protective effect of Dabigatran, Rivaroxaban and Apixaban to Wafarin (Noseworthy et al. 2016). This data supports the use of NOAC to prevent strokes as an alternative to wafarin in patients with AF and HCM. As in the general population, LAA exclusion could be considered for unsuitable long-term anticoagulation due to the risk of bleeding, although it has not specifically been evaluated in HCM patients (Holmes et al. 2009). The CHA_2DS_2-VASc commonly used for stroke risk stratification has not been validated in the HCM population and retrospective subgroup analysis of 4,821 HCM patients followed at 7 centers revealed that it had a low predictive accuracy for thromboembolism (Guttmann et al. 2015). This data supports recent consensus guidelines from the European Society of Cardiology (ESC) that advises against the use of the CHA_2DS_2-VASc score in patients with HCM and recommends lifelong anticoagulation therapy for all patients with HCM and AF, even after the first episode (Gersh et al. 2011; Authors/Task Force members et al. 2014). The prophylactic use of anticoagulants to prevent stroke in patients at high risk of AF but in whom no arrhythmia has been detected has not yet been investigated or recommended. Frequent rhythm screening is required.

Pharmacological Treatment

The relative benefit of rhythm versus rate control in the management of AF in HCM remains uncertain. However, for the majority of HCM patients, AF results in a symptomatic decline requiring restoration and maintenance of sinus rhythm, especially in case of rapid ventricular rate or LVOT obstruction. Despite the lack of randomized controlled trials comparing antiarrhythmic drug therapy to catheter ablation procedures, guidelines favour antiarrhythmic medications as a first line to prevent long-term recurrence of AF (Gersh et al. 2011; Authors/Task Force members et al. 2014).

Amiodarone is the least pro-arrhythmic and most effective drug at preventing AF recurrence. It is recommended following DC cardioversion (Class IIa, LOE B) by the 2014 ESC guidelines on HCM (Authors/Task Force members et al. 2014). However, its potential toxicity limits its use in young patients. The minimum effective dose should be employed and careful surveillance for thyroid, hepatic, pulmonary and neurologic toxicity should be implemented. Disopyramide is used to treat LVOT obstruction but its effects on AF suppression in HCM is unknown. It is often used in young patients as an alternative to amiodarone due to its toxicity. Disopyramide's negative inotropic effect restricts its use on LVOT obstruction patients, in association with a concomitant AV node blocking agent, as it can accelerate AV nodal conduction. QT prolongation and risk of anticholinergic or pro-arrhythmic effects require close monitoring during drug titration. Finally, although not as effective, sotalol is often used as a first line antiarrhythmic therapy in order to avoid the side effects caused by amiodarone or disopyramide. A prolonged QT interval and pro-arrhythmic risk both require careful monitoring. Flecainide or propafenone are generally avoided owing to concerns about pro-arrhythmic effects and haemodynamic impairement. Significant clinical experience with dronedarone is lacking, and it is not recommended in HCM (Camm et al. 2012).

When maintenance of sinus rhythm is not deemed feasible, rate control strategy remains the only option. In preserved LVEF patients, various beta-blockers and verapamil or diltiazem can be used to achieve a resting rate < 100 BPM without symptomatic bradycardia. In the presence of systolic dysfunction, the therapeutic choice is limited to bisoprolol or carvedilol. Digoxin is a positive inotropic agent that can exacerbate the LVOT gradient. Therefore, its use for chronic AF rate control, alone or in combination with beta-blockers, is restricted in HCM to the subgroup with advanced LV dysfunction (Gersh et al. 2011; Authors/Task Force members et al. 2014). The adequacy of rate control should be assessed during exercise.

When pharmacological rate control is ineffective or not tolerated, AV node ablation with pacemaker insertion may be indicated. Information about the long-term effects of RV pacing on LV function in HCM patients is lacking. Therefore, the choice of pacing should be in line with ESC guidelines, with the exception that resynchronisation therapy may be considered in patients with LVEF <50% (Camm et al. 2012).

AF Ablation

To date, no randomised controlled trials comparing AF catheter ablation to medical therapy have been done in HCM. Small series of AF ablated patients have shown that the acute and late success rate of the ablation is nearly two-fold lower than in lone AF, requiring more redo procedures, and more antiarrhythmic drugs during follow-up (Providencia et al. 2016; Derejko et al. 2013). Complication rates are similar to those observed in large RF ablation series (Providencia et al. 2016; Bassiouny et al. 2015; Cappato et al. 2010; Shah et al. 2012), but heart failure and congestive symptoms may increase postablation hospitalisation stays and readmission rates at 30 days (Contreras-Valdes et al. 2015). In a meta-analysis of 5 observational studies of radiofrequency catheter ablation with a median follow-up of 1.8 years, freedom from atrial arrhythmias was only 38.7% in the HCM group compared to 49.8% in the control group. With more than one procedure, success rate remained lower in the HCM group (51.8%) than in the control (71.2%). Chances of remaining on antiarrhythmic drugs following a successful ablation were fivefold higher in patients with HCM compared to the control group. Finally, overall efficacy of AF ablation in HCM was at least 50% lower than in the controls for more than one procedure (Providencia et al. 2016). Considering the limited efficacy of antiarrhythmic drugs over time, the specific substrate of HCM, the fact that ablation was performed late in the course of the disease (median 5.9 years after the diagnosis of atrial arrhythmia) and the greater part (more than 50% in half of the studies) of non-paroxysmal AF included, a 52% success rate after a median of 1.4 procedures seems nevertheless remarkable.

Not surprisingly, LA size and AF type are the greatest predictors of procedural success identified. Others factors include age, NYHA class, LA pressure, LVOT obstruction and AF duration in months. This may have implications for an early and aggressive rhythm control strategy using catheter ablation in younger patients with a shorter duration of AF and less dilated atria. In the general population, adverse atrial remodeling is correlated to AF duration and has been proven to be a major factor of AF recurrence after ablation (Hussein et al. 2016). Effective AF ablation with a negligible AF burden over 12 months is associated with significant reverse structural remodeling (Walters et al. 2016). This factor may be of significant importance in HCM where progressive atrial remodeling plays a major role, even in the absence of AF. At present, AF ablation in HCM patients is still limited in the guidelines to patients very symptomatic under medical treatment or who are unable to take antiarrhythmic drugs (Authors/Task Force members et al. 2014). However technical issues in ablation strategy need to be clarified: whether radiofrequency energy is the optimal energy source (versus other sources such as cryo-energy) and whether pulmonary vein isolation and targeting sustained atrial tachycardias is superior to a more extensive approach beyond PV isolation (linear lines, posterior wall isolation, targeting complex fractionated electrograms, rotors, ganglionic plexi and non-PV triggers).

There is limited data suggesting that surgical ablation of AF in HCM is both effective and safe (Bassiouny et al. 2015; Lapenna et al. 2017). It has been performed as a concomitant procedure in patients undergoing a surgical myomectomy but not reported as an isolated option. A stand-alone AF surgical procedure or a hybrid approach associated with left atrial appendage occlusion should benefit HCM patients and needs to be investigated.

Conclusion

In HCM, the occurrence of AF is a turning point in the evolution of the disease, leading to an increased risk of stroke or mortality. Lifelong antithrombotic therapy is recommended after the first AF episode. Repeated screening for AF occurrence in patients with LA dilatation using connected tools may be a valuable strategy to prevent ischemic events. Poor long-term efficacy, proarrhythmic risk, as well as amiodarone toxicity all limit the long-term use of antiarrhythmic treatment in young patients. Catheter or surgical ablation might improve the course of the disease in younger patients with a shorter duration of AF and a less dilated atria, and should be evaluated for this specific population.

References

Authors/Task Force members, Perry M. Elliott, Aris Anastasakis, Michael A. Borger, Martin Borggrefe, Franco Cecchi, Philippe Charron, et al. 2014. "2014 ESC Guidelines on Diagnosis and Management of Hypertrophic Cardiomyopathy: The Task Force for the Diagnosis and Management of Hypertrophic Cardiomyopathy of the European Society of Cardiology (ESC)". *European Heart Journal* 35 (39): 2733‑79. doi:10.1093/eurheartj/ehu284.

Azarbal, Farnaz, Maneesh Singh, Gherardo Finocchiaro, Vy-Van Le, Ingela Schnittger, Paul Wang, Jonathan Myers, Euan Ashley, et Marco Perez. 2014. "Exercise Capacity and Paroxysmal Atrial Fibrillation in Patients with Hypertrophic Cardiomyopathy." *Heart (British Cardiac Society)* 100 (8): 624‑30. doi:10.1136/heartjnl-2013-304908.

Bassiouny, Mohamed, Bruce D. Lindsay, Harry Lever, Walid Saliba, Allan Klein, Moustafa Banna, JoEllyn Abraham, et al. 2015. "Outcomes of Nonpharmacologic Treatment of Atrial Fibrillation in Patients with Hypertrophic Cardiomyopathy." *Heart Rhythm* 12 (7): 1438‑47. doi:10.1016/j.hrthm.2015.03.042.

Camm, A. John, Gregory Y. H. Lip, Raffaele De Caterina, Irene Savelieva, Dan Atar, Stefan H. Hohnloser, Gerhard Hindricks, Paulus Kirchhof, et ESC Committee for Practice Guidelines (CPG). 2012. "2012 Focused Update of the ESC Guidelines for the Management of Atrial Fibrillation: An Update of the 2010 ESC Guidelines for the Management of Atrial Fibrillation. Developed with the Special Contribution of the European Heart Rhythm Association." *European Heart Journal* 33 (21): 2719‑47. doi:10.1093/eurheartj/ehs253.

Cappato, Riccardo, Hugh Calkins, Shih-Ann Chen, Wyn Davies, Yoshito Iesaka, Jonathan Kalman, You-Ho Kim, et al. 2010. "Updated Worldwide Survey on the Methods, Efficacy, and Safety of Catheter Ablation for Human Atrial Fibrillation." *Circulation. Arrhythmia and Electrophysiology* 3 (1): 32‑38. doi:10.1161/CIRCEP.109.859116.

Contreras-Valdes, Fernando M., Alfred E. Buxton, Mark E. Josephson, et Elad Anter. 2015. "Atrial Fibrillation Ablation in Patients with Hypertrophic Cardiomyopathy: Long-Term Outcomes and Clinical Predictors." *Journal of the American College of Cardiology* 65 (14): 1485‑87. doi:10.1016/j.jacc.2014.12.063.

Debonnaire, Philippe, Emer Joyce, Yasmine Hiemstra, Bart J. Mertens, Douwe E. Atsma, Martin J. Schalij, Jeroen J. Bax, Victoria Delgado, et Nina Ajmone Marsan. 2017. "Left Atrial Size and Function in Hypertrophic Cardiomyopathy Patients and Risk of New-Onset Atrial Fibrillation." *Circulation. Arrhythmia and Electrophysiology* 10 (2). doi:10.1161/CIRCEP.116.004052.

Derejko, Paweł, Magdalena Polańska, Lidia Chojnowska, Ilona Michałowska, Anna Wójcik, Ewa Piotrowicz, Agnieszka Lech, et al. 2013. "Catheter Ablation of Atrial Fibrillation in Patients with Hypertrophic Cardiomyopathy: Atrial Fibrillation Type Determines the Success Rate." *Kardiologia Polska* 71 (1): 17‑24.

Eleid, Mackram F., Tomas Konecny, Marek Orban, Partho P. Sengupta, Virend K. Somers, James M. Parish, Farouk Mookadam, et al. 2009. "High Prevalence of Abnormal Nocturnal Oximetry in Patients with Hypertrophic Cardiomyopathy." *Journal of the American College of Cardiology* 54 (19): 1805‑9. doi:10.1016/j.jacc.2009.07.030.

Gersh, Bernard J., Barry J. Maron, Robert O. Bonow, Joseph A. Dearani, Michael A. Fifer, Mark S. Link, Srihari S. Naidu, et al. 2011. "2011 ACCF/AHA Guideline for the Diagnosis and Treatment of Hypertrophic Cardiomyopathy: A Report of the American College of Cardiology Foundation/American Heart Association Task Force on Practice Guidelines. Developed in Collaboration with the American Association for Thoracic Surgery, American Society of Echocardiography, American Society of Nuclear Cardiology, Heart Failure Society of America, Heart Rhythm Society, Society for Cardiovascular Angiography and Interventions, and Society of Thoracic Surgeons." *Journal of the American College of Cardiology* 58 (25): e212-260. doi:10.1016/j.jacc.2011.06.011.

Gruver, E. J., D. Fatkin, G. A. Dodds, J. Kisslo, B. J. Maron, J. G. Seidman, et C. E. Seidman. 1999. "Familial Hypertrophic Cardiomyopathy and Atrial Fibrillation Caused by Arg663His Beta-Cardiac Myosin Heavy Chain Mutation." *The American Journal of Cardiology* 83 (12A): 13H‑18H.

Guttmann, Oliver P., Menelaos Pavlou, Constantinos O'Mahony, Lorenzo Monserrat, Aristides Anastasakis, Claudio Rapezzi, Elena Biagini, et al. 2015. "Prediction of Thrombo-Embolic Risk in Patients with Hypertrophic Cardiomyopathy (HCM Risk-CVA)." *European Journal of Heart Failure* 17 (8): 837‑45. doi:10.1002/ejhf.316.

Holmes, David R., Vivek Y. Reddy, Zoltan G. Turi, Shephal K. Doshi, Horst Sievert, Maurice Buchbinder, Christopher M. Mullin, Peter Sick, et PROTECT AF Investigators. 2009. "Percutaneous Closure of the Left Atrial Appendage versus Warfarin Therapy for Prevention of Stroke in Patients with Atrial Fibrillation: A Randomised Non-Inferiority Trial." *Lancet (London, England)* 374 (9689): 534‑42. doi:10.1016/S0140-6736(09)61343-X.

Hussein, Ayman A., Walid I. Saliba, Amr Barakat, Mohammed Bassiouny, Mohammed Chamsi-Pasha, Rasha Al-Bawardy, Ali Hakim, et al. 2016. "Radiofrequency Ablation of Persistent Atrial Fibrillation: Diagnosis-to-Ablation Time, Markers of Pathways of Atrial Remodeling, and Outcomes." *Circulation. Arrhythmia and Electrophysiology* 9 (1): e003669. doi:10.1161/CIRCEP.115.003669.

Lapenna, Elisabetta, Alberto Pozzoli, Michele De Bonis, Giovanni La Canna, Teodora Nisi, Simona Nascimbene, Luca Vicentini, et al. 2017. "Mid-Term Outcomes of Concomitant Surgical Ablation of Atrial Fibrillation in Patients Undergoing Cardiac Surgery for Hypertrophic Cardiomyopathy†." *European Journal of Cardio-Thoracic Surgery: Official Journal of the European Association for Cardio-Thoracic Surgery* 51 (6): 1112- 18. doi:10.1093/ejcts/ezx017.

Lee, Sang-Eun, Jin-Kyu Park, Jae-Sun Uhm, Jong Youn Kim, Hui-Nam Pak, Moon-Hyoung Lee, et Boyoung Joung. 2017. "Impact of Atrial Fibrillation on the Clinical Course of Apical Hypertrophic Cardiomyopathy." *Heart (British Cardiac Society)* 103 (19): 1496- 1501. doi:10.1136/heartjnl-2016-310720.

MacIntyre, Ciorsti, et Neal K. Lakdawala. 2016. "Management of Atrial Fibrillation in Hypertrophic Cardiomyopathy." *Circulation* 133 (19): 1901- 5. doi:10.1161/CIRCULATIONAHA.115.015085.

Maron, Barry J. 2002. "Hypertrophic Cardiomyopathy: A Systematic Review." *JAMA* 287 (10): 1308- 20.

Maron, Barry J., Steve R. Ommen, Christopher Semsarian, Paolo Spirito, Iacopo Olivotto, et Martin S. Maron. 2014. "Hypertrophic Cardiomyopathy: Present and Future, with Translation into Contemporary Cardiovascular Medicine." *Journal of the American College of Cardiology* 64 (1): 83- 99. doi:10.1016/j.jacc.2014.05.003.

Masri, Ahmad, Mohamed Kanj, Maran Thamilarasan, Oussama Wazni, Nicholas G. Smedira, Harry M. Lever, et Milind Y. Desai. 2017. "Outcomes in Hypertrophic Cardiomyopathy Patients with and without Atrial Fibrillation: A Survival Meta-Analysis." *Cardiovascular Diagnosis and Therapy* 7 (1): 36- 44. doi:10.21037/cdt.2016.11.23.

Noseworthy, Peter A., Xiaoxi Yao, Nilay D. Shah, et Bernard J. Gersh. 2016. "Stroke and Bleeding Risks in NOAC- and Warfarin-Treated Patients With Hypertrophic Cardiomyopathy and Atrial Fibrillation." *Journal of the American College of Cardiology* 67 (25): 3020‐21. doi:10.1016/j.jacc.2016.04.026.

Olivotto, I., F. Cecchi, S. A. Casey, A. Dolara, J. H. Traverse, et B. J. Maron. 2001. "Impact of Atrial Fibrillation on the Clinical Course of Hypertrophic Cardiomyopathy." *Circulation* 104 (21): 2517‐24.

Owens, David S. 2014. "Hypertrophic Cardiomyopathy: Exercising a Strategy of Personalised Medicine." *Heart (British Cardiac Society)* 100 (8): 603‐4. doi:10.1136/heartjnl-2013-305154.

Park, Kyoung-Min, Sung Il Im, Eun Kyoung Kim, Sang-Chol Lee, Seung-Jung Park, June Soo Kim, et Young Keun On. 2016. "Atrial Fibrillation in Hypertrophic Cardiomyopathy: Is the Extent of Septal Hypertrophy Important?" *PloS One* 11 (6): e0156410. doi:10.1371/journal.pone.0156410.

Providencia, Rui, Perry Elliott, Kiran Patel, Jack McCready, Girish Babu, Neil Srinivasan, Kostantinos Bronis, et al. 2016. "Catheter Ablation for Atrial Fibrillation in Hypertrophic Cardiomyopathy: A Systematic Review and Meta-Analysis." *Heart (British Cardiac Society)* 102 (19): 1533‐43. doi:10.1136/heartjnl-2016-309406.

Rowin, Ethan J., Alexander Orfanos, N. A. Mark Estes, Wendy Wang, Mark S. Link, Martin S. Maron, et Barry J. Maron. 2017. "Occurrence and Natural History of Clinically Silent Episodes of Atrial Fibrillation in Hypertrophic Cardiomyopathy." *The American Journal of Cardiology* 119 (11): 1862‐65. doi:10.1016/j.amjcard.2017.02.040.

Shah, Rashmee U., James V. Freeman, David Shilane, Paul J. Wang, Alan S. Go, et Mark A. Hlatky. 2012. "Procedural Complications, Rehospitalizations, and Repeat Procedures after Catheter Ablation for Atrial Fibrillation." *Journal of the American College of Cardiology* 59 (2): 143‐49. doi:10.1016/j.jacc.2011.08.068.

Siontis, Konstantinos C., Jeffrey B. Geske, Kevin Ong, Rick A. Nishimura, Steve R. Ommen, et Bernard J. Gersh. 2014. "Atrial Fibrillation in Hypertrophic Cardiomyopathy: Prevalence, Clinical Correlations, and

Mortality in a Large High-Risk Population." *Journal of the American Heart Association* 3 (3): e001002. doi:10.1161/JAHA.114.001002.

Steinberg, Jonathan S., Niraj Varma, Iwona Cygankiewicz, Peter Aziz, Paweł Balsam, Adrian Baranchuk, Daniel J. Cantillon, et al. 2017. "2017 ISHNE-HRS Expert Consensus Statement on Ambulatory ECG and External Cardiac Monitoring/Telemetry." *Heart Rhythm* 14 (7): e55 - 96. doi:10.1016/j.hrthm.2017.03.038.

Tuluce, Kamil, et Selcen Yakar Tuluce. 2015. "Predictors of Atrial Fibrillation Risk in Hypertrophic Cardiomyopathy." *Journal of Atrial Fibrillation* 7 (5): 1200. doi:10.4022/jafib.1200.

Vaidya, Kaivan, Christopher Semsarian, et Kim H. Chan. 2017. "Atrial Fibrillation in Hypertrophic Cardiomyopathy." *Heart, Lung & Circulation* 26 (9): 975 - 82. doi:10.1016/j.hlc.2017.05.116.

Velzen, Hannah G. van, Dominic A. M. J. Theuns, Sing-Chien Yap, Michelle Michels, et Arend F. L. Schinkel. 2017. "Incidence of Device-Detected Atrial Fibrillation and Long-Term Outcomes in Patients With Hypertrophic Cardiomyopathy." *The American Journal of Cardiology* 119 (1): 100 - 105. doi:10.1016/j.amjcard.2016.08.092.

Walters, Tomos E., Ashley Nisbet, Gwilym M. Morris, Gabriel Tan, Megan Mearns, Eliza Teo, Nigel Lewis, et al. 2016. "Progression of Atrial Remodeling in Patients with High-Burden Atrial Fibrillation: Implications for Early Ablative Intervention." *Heart Rhythm* 13 (2): 331 - 39. doi:10.1016/j.hrthm.2015.10.028.

Wilke, Iris, Katrin Witzel, Julia Münch, Simon Pecha, Stephan Blankenberg, Hermann Reichenspurner, Stephan Willems, Monica Patten, et Ali Aydin. 2016. "High Incidence of De Novo and Subclinical Atrial Fibrillation in Patients with Hypertrophic Cardiomyopathy and Cardiac Rhythm Management Device." *Journal of Cardiovascular Electrophysiology* 27 (7): 779 - 84. doi:10.1111/jce.12982.

In: Hypertrophic Cardiomyopathy
Editor: Ikram Kammoun ISBN: 978-1-53613-003-4

Chapter 4

MITRAL VALVE ABNORMALITIES IDENTIFIED BY CARDIAC MAGNETIC RESONANCE IN PATIENTS WITH HYPERTROPHIED CARDIOMYOPATHY

Henda Neji**, MD, Monia Attia, MD,
Saoussen Hantous-Zannad, MD, Ines Baccouche, MD and Khaoula Ben Miled M'rad, MD
Imaging Department, Tunis ElManar University, Tunis, Tunisia

ABSTRACT

Abnormal myocardium thickening is the hallmark of hypertrophic cardiomyopathy. Mitral valve abnormalities are among the most important features that may accompany or precede this thickening in patients with positive genotype – negative phenotype. The abnormalities were first assessed by cardiac catheterization and then by ultrasonography. Now, magnetic resonance imaging (MRI) provides a detailed description of them and their functional impact, making it possible to better plan their management.

In this chapter, MRI exploration protocol and abnormal morphological and functional mitral apparatus features are described.

* Corresponding author: hendaneji@gmail.com.

Keywords: hypertrophic cardiomyopathy, mitral valve apparatus, MRI

Introduction

Diagnosis of Hypertrophied cardiomyopathy (HCM) is classically based on abnormal myocardium thickening in the absence of a sufficient hemodynamic explanation for hypertrophy. However, this can occur late in life and it has been demonstrated that it can be preceded by other morphological changes, some of which involve the mitral valve apparatus (MVA) (Schantz et al., 2016). Its intrinsic and functional abnormalities are common in patients with HCM, accounting for about 70% in autopsy studies. They are mostly observed in cases of septal thickening with left ventricle outflow tract (LVOT) obstruction. They should be carefully identified as they may require surgical management (K Kaple et al., 2008).

Advances in imaging techniques, particularly in cardiac magnetic resonance (CMR), have made it possible to understand the complex interaction between all MVA abnormalities and their dynamic impact thanks to its high spatial and temporal resolution (Cavalcante, S Barboza, and Lever 2012; Dulguerov et al., 2016; Maron et al., 2011).

CMR Protocol

To evaluate the MVA in HCM, CMR protocol should include (Tarkiainen et al., 2016; Morant et al., 2017):

- Cine sequences in short axis, 4 chamber-, 3 chamber- and 2 chamber- views for morphological analysis of the MVA, leaflet measurements as well as dynamic evaluation of blood flow in the LVOT and through the mitral valve. They can also assess left ventricle (LV) function and mass as well as papillary muscles (PM) mass.
- Phase contrast exploration of the LVOT to evaluate the obstruction gradient.

– First pass perfusion and late gadolinium enhancement sequences are performed to assess microvascular abnormalities and fibrosis in whole myocardium.

Normal Anatomy of the Mitral Valve Apparatus

Normal MV leaflets have a convexo-concave line of closure joining their commissures. Anterior and posterior leaflets do not exceed 30 and 15mm, respectively. A normal left ventricle contains 2 PM attaching to the middle third of the posterior wall and arising from the trabeculae carneae. The anterolateral PM usually has a single head whereas the posteromedial has two. Accessory PM can be found in 15% of the normal population (Silbiger 2016).

Mitral Valve Apparatus Abnormalities

MVA abnormalities are well assessed by CMR. They include morphological and functional modifications.

Elongation of Mitral Valve Leaflets

Elongation of MV leaflets is the most studied and documented abnormality in the literature. One or both leaflets can be involved. Four theories explain the elongation: sarcomere gene mutation, stretch effect, concomitant familial MV disease, and paracrine effects from the adjacent hypertrophic ventricle (Cavalcante, S Barboza, and Lever 2012). Leaflet elongation has been observed early on both in subjects who have an HCM-associated mutation but who have not yet developed thickening as well as in pediatric patients with HCM, suggesting that mitral elongation is a primary phenotypic expression of HCM and is not acquired due to stretch from systolic anterior motion (SAM) (Cavalcante, S Barboza, and Lever 2012; Sherrid et al., 2016; Maron et al., 2011; Schantz et al. 2016).

Elongated leaflets are not myxomatous (Sherrid et al., 2016). Propagation and worsening of elongation is explained by the Venturi effect: the mitral valve is attracted towards the septum by high blood velocity resulting from increased ventricular function in a narrowed outflow tract (Hagège et al., 2011).

MRI measures MV leaflets with good reproducibility. Leaflets are measured in mid- or end- diastole three chamber view (Maron et al., 2011; Hagège et al., 2011). The length is defined as the distance between the tips and the posterior aortic wall for the anterior one and to the basal LV free wall for the posterior one (Maron et al., 2011; Hagège et al., 2011). Demarcation between chordae and leaflet tip is made visually by inspecting cine images (Maron et al., 2011; Hagège et al., 2011; Morant et al., 2017) (Figure 1).

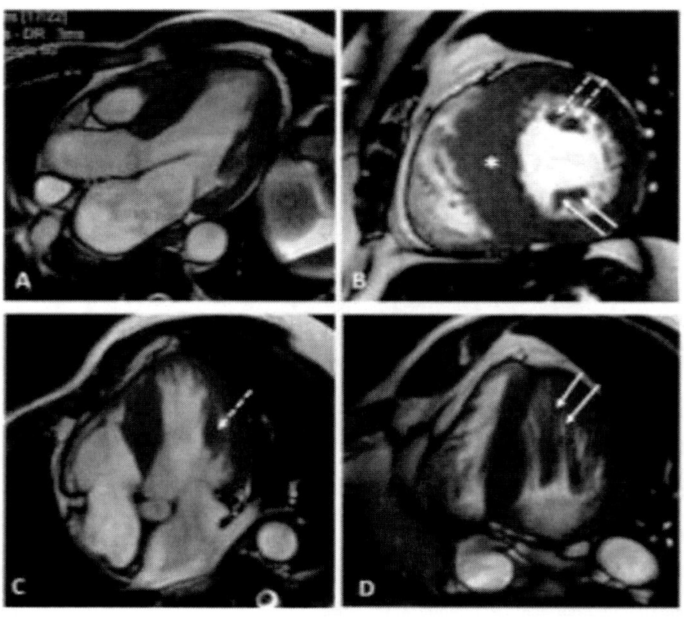

Figure 1. CMR in a patient with HCM.
-A: three chambers view showing elongation of both leaflets of the MV
-B: short axis view, C and D: 4 chambers view showing interventricular septum hypertrophy (asterisk), double anterolateral PM anteriorly displaced (arrows) and bifid posterolateral PM (dashed arrow).

MV leaflets in patients with HCM are 1.5 to 1.7 cm longer than in normal patients. A CMR study of 172 patients comparing patients with HCM and normal patients showed that anterior and posterior leaflet length was 26 ± 5 versus 19 ± 5 mm and 14 ± 4 versus 10 ± 3 mm, respectively (Maron et al., 2011).

Leaflets coapt in the central part rather than in the tips (Cavalcante, S Barboza, and Lever 2012). Coaptation occurs with a mean of 26 mm under the annulus plane rather than 14 mm (Sherrid et al., 2016). Long MV leaflets and protrusion participate in SAM genesis and LVOT obstruction during exercise (Sherrid et al., 2016; Henein et al., 2016). The coaptation point of the mitral leaflets is closer to the septum. Maximal and mean tenting time are higher in patients with HCM with SAM than that of controls (Hagège et al., 2011).

Leaflet elongation correlates with the degree of septal hypertrophy and with obstructive HCM but does not correlate with LV mass index or maximal wall thickness (K Kaple et al., 2008; Maron et al., 2011; Sherrid et al., 2016).

Papillary Muscle Anomalies

CMR, due to its high spatial and temporal resolution, offers a detailed assessment of anterior and posterior PMs (number, location, mobility and attachments). They are well assessed in four- and two- chamber views, respectively (Cavalcante, S Barboza, and Lever 2012; Silbiger 2016; Teo, Teoh, and Hung 2015). Primary PM Abnormalities include hypertrophy, anterior displacement, anomalous insertion and accessory papillary muscles (Figures 1 and 2) (Teo, Teoh, and Hung 2015). They most frequently involve the anterolateral PM (Klues, Roberts, and Maron 1991).

Hypertrophy of PMs (defined as a combined mass $>7g/m^2$) occurs in more than half of patients (Silbiger 2016). Direct attachment to the ventricle wall or to the leaflet was observed in 13% of patients (Klues, Roberts, and Maron 1991). Anterior and apical displacement may cause mid-cavity obstruction by simple contact between the papillary muscle and the mid-septum. It is correlated with higher peak gradient and is responsible for systolic anterior motion (SAM) of the MV as well (Cavalcante, S Barboza, and Lever 2012; Sherrid et al., 2016; Klues, Roberts, and Maron 1991) (Figure 3). PMs may have a medial displacement resulting in reduction of the distance between them (Silbiger 2016). PMs may be double or bifid. Accessory PM may hypertrophy and occupy an anterior or apical position, favoring SAM occurrence (Silbiger 2016; Cavalcante, S Barboza, and Lever 2012; K Kaple et al., 2008).

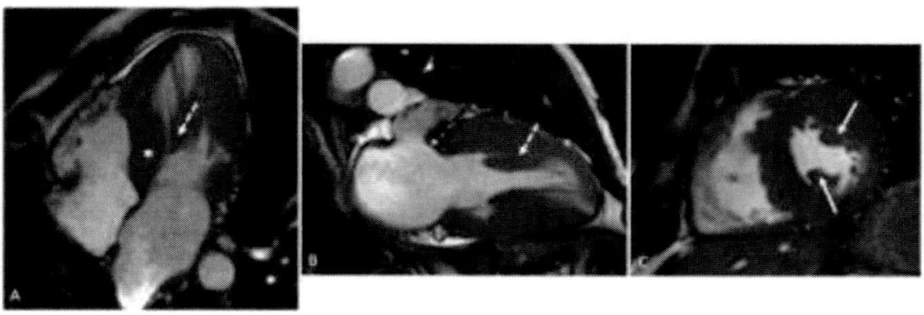

Figure 2. CMR with 4 chambers (A), 2 chambers (B) and short axis (C) cine views in diastole showing hypertrophied PMs (arrows) with anterior and apical displacement of the anterolateral PM (dashed arrows). This latter has a near contact with the interventricular septum (asterisk).

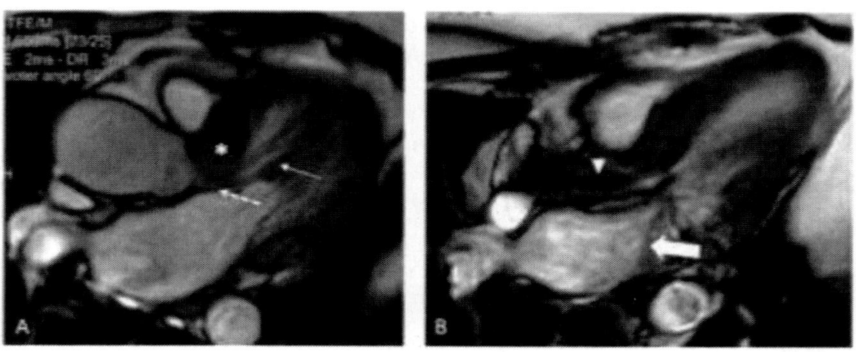

Figure 3. CMR with 3 chambers cine views showing septal hypertrophy (asterisk), direct insertion of the anterolateral PM (arrow) on the tip of the anterior leaflet which is thickened (dashed arrow). Note the narrowing and the severe obstruction of the LVOT (arrowhead) as well as mitral regurgitation (thick arrow).

Systolic Anterior Motion of the Mitral Valve

SAM was first reported as participating in LVOT obstruction in 1969 (Sherrid et al., 2016). Thirty to 60% of patients with HCM present with SAM. LVOT obstruction occurs in one-third of cases at rest (Hagège et al., 2011). In the remaining cases, dynamic LVOT obstruction should be investigated when there is no resting gradient in symptomatic patients either by exercise or by the Valsalva maneuver (Henein et al., 2016; Hagège et al., 2011). SAM is created by anterior displacement of the papillary muscle and mitral leaflets elongation even in the absence of septal hypertrophy (Hagège et al., 2011). In fact, there is posterior displacement of the flow in LVOT aligning with the free margins of the MV leaflets (Silbiger 2016). Residual leaflet portion after coaptation will interpose in the outflow pathway at the beginning of systolic ejection, which initiates SAM (Figure 4) (Hagège et al., 2011).

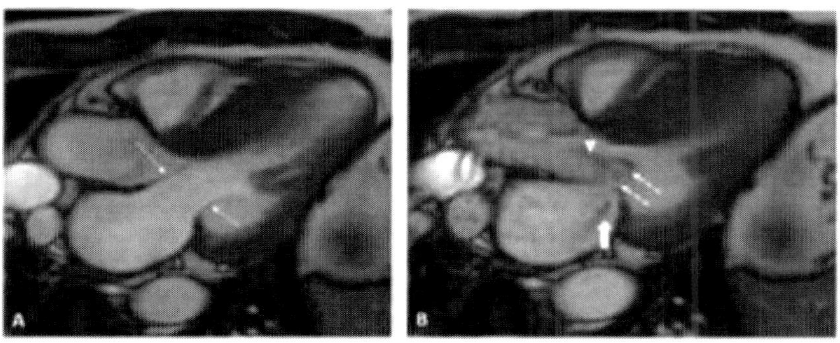

Figure 4. Three chambers cine views in diastole (A) and systole (B) showing elongated anterior and posterior leaflets (arrows). Residual posterior leaflet after coaptation (dashed arrows) interposing in the LVOT creating obstruction flow artefact (arrowhead) and mitral regurgitation (thick arrow).

Chordal Abnormalities

Mitral chordae can be fibrotic and retracted (Maron et al., 2011). They may also be ruptured.

Intrinsic Mitral Abnormalities

Intrinsic MV abnormalities include mitral annulus calcification, MV prolapse, chordal rupture, myxomatous changes as well as fibrosis and retraction of the leaflets. This latter is caused by repetitive contact with the interventricular septum in case of SAM and may accentuate mitral regurgitation (Silbiger 2016; K Kaple et al., 2008) (Figure 3).

Mitral Valve Regurgitation

Regurgitation may result from intrinsic mitral abnormalities and/or from lack of leaflet coaptation at mid-systole as well as the limitation of the posterior leaflet excursion (Cavalcante, S Barboza, and Lever 2012; Hagège et al., 2011). The mechanism of regurgitation should be well determined to accurately plan its management (Teo, Teoh, and Hung 2015). Mitral regurgitation is correlated to the degree of LVOT obstruction (Teo, Teoh, and Hung 2015).

On CMR 3- chamber view, mitral regurgitation flow caused by SAM is posterolateral and perpendicular to the flow in the LVOT (Silbiger 2016) (Figures 3 and 4).

Conclusion

Morphological MV abnormalities are likely an early phenotypic expression of HCM, the most documented of which is leaflet elongation. These abnormalities can lead to dynamic changes of the valve including SAM and regurgitation. CMR is a good non- irradiating imaging technique that can assess both types of MVA modification.

REFERENCES

Cavalcante, João, Joaquim S Barboza, and Harry Lever. 2012. "Diversity of Mitral Valve Abnormalities in Obstructive Hypertrophic Cardiomyopathy." *Progress in Cardiovascular Diseases* 54 (May): 517–22. doi:10.1016/j.pcad.2012.03.002.

Dulguerov, Filip, Cecilia Marcacci, Clara Alexandrescu, K. M. John Chan, and Gilles D. Dreyfus. 2016. "Hypertrophic Obstructive Cardiomyopathy: The Mitral Valve Could Be the Key." *European Journal of Cardio-Thoracic Surgery* 50 (1): 61–65. doi:10.1093/ejcts/ezv473.

Hagège, Albert A., Patrick Bruneval, Robert A. Levine, Michel Desnos, Hany Neamatalla, and Daniel P. Judge. 2011. "The Mitral Valve in Hypertrophic Cardiomyopathy." *Journal of Cardiovascular Translational Research* 4 (6):757–66. doi:10.1007/s12265-011-9319-6.

Henein, Michael, Sandra Arvidsson, Björn Pilebro, Christer Backman, Stellan Mörner, and Per Lindqvist. 2016. "Long Mitral Valve Leaflets Determine Left Ventricular Outflow Tract Obstruction during Exercise in Hypertrophic Cardiomyopathy." *International Journal of Cardiology* 212 (June): 47–53. doi:10.1016/j.ijcard.2016.03.041.

K. Kaple, Ryan, Ross Murphy, Linda M DiPaola, Penny Houghtaling, Harry Lever, Bruce W Lytle, Eugene Blackstone, and Nicholas G Smedira. 2008. "Mitral Valve Abnormalities in Hypertrophic Cardiomyopathy: Echocardiographic Features and Surgical Outcomes." *The Annals of Thoracic Surgery* 85 (June): 1527–35, 1535.e1. doi:10.1016/j.athoracsur.2008.01.061.

Klues, H. G., W. C. Roberts, and B. J. Maron. 1991. "Anomalous Insertion of Papillary Muscle Directly into Anterior Mitral Leaflet in Hypertrophic Cardiomyopathy. Significance in Producing Left Ventricular Outflow Obstruction." *Circulation* 84 (3): 1188–97.

Maron, Martin S., Iacopo Olivotto, Caitlin Harrigan, Evan Appelbaum, C. Michael Gibson, John R. Lesser, Tammy S. Haas, James E. Udelson, Warren J. Manning, and Barry J. Maron. 2011. "Mitral Valve Abnormalities Identified by Cardiovascular Magnetic Resonance

Represent a Primary Phenotypic Expression of Hypertrophic CardiomyopathyClinical Perspective." *Circulation* 124 (1): 40–47. doi:10.1161/CIRCULATIONAHA.110.985812.

Morant, Kareem, Yoko Mikami, Immaculate Nevis, David McCarty, John Stirrat, David Scholl, Martin Rajchl, et al., 2017. "Contribution of Mitral Valve Leaflet Length and Septal Wall Thickness to Outflow Tract Obstruction in Patients with Hypertrophic Cardiomyopathy." *The International Journal of Cardiovascular Imaging* 33 (8): 1201–11. doi:10.1007/s10554-017-1103-5.

Schantz, Daryl, Lee Benson, Jonathan Windram, Derek Wong, Andreea Dragulescu, Shi-Joon Yoo, Luc Mertens, Mark Friedberg, Bahiyah Al Nafisi, and Lars Grosse-Wortmann. 2016. "Abnormal Mitral Valve Dimensions in Pediatric Patients with Hypertrophic Cardiomyopathy." *Pediatric Cardiology* 37 (4): 784–88. doi:10.1007/s00246-016-1351-5.

Sherrid, Mark V., Sandhya Balaram, Bette Kim, Leon Axel, and Daniel G. Swistel. 2016. "The Mitral Valve in Obstructive Hypertrophic Cardiomyopathy: A Test in Context." *Journal of the American College of Cardiology* 67 (15): 1846–58. doi:10.1016/j.jacc.2016.01.071.

Silbiger, Jeffrey J. 2016. "Abnormalities of the Mitral Apparatus in Hypertrophic Cardiomyopathy: Echocardiographic, Pathophysiologic, and Surgical Insights." *Journal of the American Society of Echocardiography: Official Publication of the American Society of Echocardiography* 29 (7): 622–39. doi:10.1016/j.echo.2016.03.003.

Tarkiainen, Mika, Petri Sipola, Mikko Jalanko, Tiina Heliö, Mika Laine, Vesa Järvinen, Kaisu Häyrinen, Kirsi Lauerma, and Johanna Kuusisto. 2016. "Cardiovascular Magnetic Resonance of Mitral Valve Length in Hypertrophic Cardiomyopathy." *Journal of Cardiovascular Magnetic Resonance* 18 (December). doi:10.1186/s12968-016-0250-5.

Teo, Eliza P., Jonathan G. Teoh, and Judy Hung. 2015. "Mitral Valve and Papillary Muscle Abnormalities in Hypertrophic Obstructive Cardiomyopathy." *Current Opinion in Cardiology* 30 (5): 475–482. doi:10.1097/HCO.0000000000000200.

In: Hypertrophic Cardiomyopathy
Editor: Ikram Kammoun
ISBN: 978-1-53613-003-4

Chapter 5

ECHOCARDIOGRAPHIC PREDICTORS OF UNFAVOURABLE OUTCOME IN HYPERTROPHIC CARDIOMYOPATHY

Ikram Kammoun**[*], **MD, Sonia Marrakchi, MD, Emna Bennour, MD and Salem Kachboura, MD
Department of cardiology, Tunis ElManar University, Ariana, Tunisia

ABSTRACT

Hypertrophic cardiomyopathy is the most frequent genetic cardiomyopathy, characterized by marked variability in morphological expression.

Prognostic evaluation and stratification of sudden cardiac death in these patients is difficult because of the high variability of the natural history.

Some variables predicting poor prognosis have been reported over the last few years (severe left ventricular hypertrophy, left atrial dilatation, severe obstruction, midventricular obstruction, apical aneurysm, left ventricular dysfunction and strain parameters) and are easily identifiable with echocardiography.

[*] Corresponding author: kammounikram@yahoo.fr.

These parameters and their prognostic value are detailed in this chapter.

Keywords: hypertrophic cardiomyopathy, death, echocardiography

INTRODUCTION

Hypertrophic cardiomyopathy is the most frequent genetic cardiomyopathy, characterized by marked variability in morphological expression.

Fifty years after Teare's description of HCM, identifying patients at high risk for sudden death remains a challenge.

The major obstacles to developing accurate prediction factors are the complexity and variability of the arrhythmogenic substrate in patients with HCM (Dimitrow et al. 2010).

None of the existing risk factors alone reliably predicts the risk of sudden cardiac death (SCD). Evaluating HCM patients requires the use of combined information (Marian 2010).

Echocardiography can thus identify some variables which will be detailed further in this chapter.

LEFT ATRIAL DILATION AND FUNCTION

A positive association was found between left atrial (LA) size and SCD in patients with HCM (O'Mahony et al. 2014; Paolo Spirito et al. 2009).

The presence of a left atrial index > 25 mm/m^2 and a left atrial diameter > 45 mm were predictive of mortality (P. Spirito and Maron 1987).

This LA diameter was recently introduced within the seven parameters of the new SCD risk prediction model (HCM Risk-SCD). This score was validated in a multicentre, retrospective, longitudinal study of 3675 patients (O'Mahony et al. 2014).

Although LA enlargement as assessed from linear dimensions was shown to independently predict long-term prognosis in HCM, it is important to recognize that this chamber frequently remodels asymmetrically and linear dimensions do not reflect true LA size.

To quantify LA size, the American Society of Echocardiography/EAE recommends that LA volume (derived from biplane area length or method of disks) be indexed to body surface area (normal indexed LA volume = 22 $\pm$ 6 ml/m^2) (Lang et al. 2015).

Losi (Losi et al. 2009) evaluated the prognostic role of LA volume in HCM by measuring LA volume at baseline and during follow-up in 140 patients.

In those patients with an enlarged LA volume (>27 mL/m^2), there was an increased risk for unfavorable outcome, defined as occurrence of sudden death, heart transplantation, or invasive reduction of obstruction.

In addition, LA volume dilated at baseline and fast dilating LA volume (volume increased more than 3 mL per year) were both independent predictors of unfavorable outcome development (odds ratio: 11.4).

This finding was confirmed in a large study (427 patients with HCM) by Hiemstra (Hiemstra et al. 2017) which demonstrated that indexed LA volume was independently associated with adverse outcome (all-cause mortality, heart transplantation, sudden cardiac death, and appropriate implantable cardioverter defibrillator therapy).

In this study, patients with an indexed LA volume $\geq$34 ml/m^2 had a worse outcome than those with <34 ml/m^2.

LA volume is largely determined by the presence of diastolic dysfunction, mitral regurgitation, and atrial myopathy with increased atrial fibrosis. This LA enlargement has consistently been identified as a strong predictor of AF development in HCM patients.

Patients who develop AF are known to have a worse prognosis of impaired exercise tolerance, hospitalization for heart failure, and higher mortality.

LA volume and function (as measured by LA strain) are independently related to new-onset AF in HCM patients.

Both LA volume (≥37 mL/m²) and strain (≤23.4%) can improve prediction of new-onset AF in patients with HCM, particularly in the subgroup with preserved LA diameter (<45mm), and may therefore be preferred over diameter for risk stratification (Debonnaire et al. 2017).

Left Ventricular Hypertrophy

In patients with HCM, the rate of sudden death increases progressively in direct relation to maximum left ventricular wall thickness, mostly when that thickness is >20 mm (P. M. Elliott et al. 2001; Sorajja et al. 2006).

This risk factor is of more prognostic significance in the younger patient.

In addition, both the severity and extent of LVH measured by transthoracic echocardiography are associated with the risk of SCD, the incidence of sudden death nearly doubled for each 5 mm increase in wall thickness.

Several studies (O'Mahony et al. 2014; P. Spirito et al. 2000; Dimitrow et al. 2010; Louie and Maron 1986) have shown the greatest risk of SCD in patients with a massive hypertrophy ≥30 mm (Figure 1) but not a lot of data exists for patients with extreme hypertrophy (≥35 mm).

Patients with a wall thickness >30 mm had a substantial long-term risk of sudden death: 20% at 10 years and 40% at 20 years (P. Spirito et al. 2000).

However, in Elliott's study (P. M. Elliott et al. 2001), an excellent survival rate was found in 40% of patients with a wall thickness of 30 mm or more but who had no other clinical risk factors. These authors concluded that a wall thickness of this magnitude cannot by itself be used as justification for implantation of an ICD in patients with HCM.

Recently, O'Mahony C. (O'Mahony et al. 2014) proposed a novel clinical risk prediction model for sudden cardiac death in hypertrophic cardiomyopathy, including the magnitude of hypertrophy.

In this HCM Risk-SCD model, compared with the risk stratification models proposed by the older guidelines, LVWT is no longer regarded as dichotomous, but as a continuous variable.

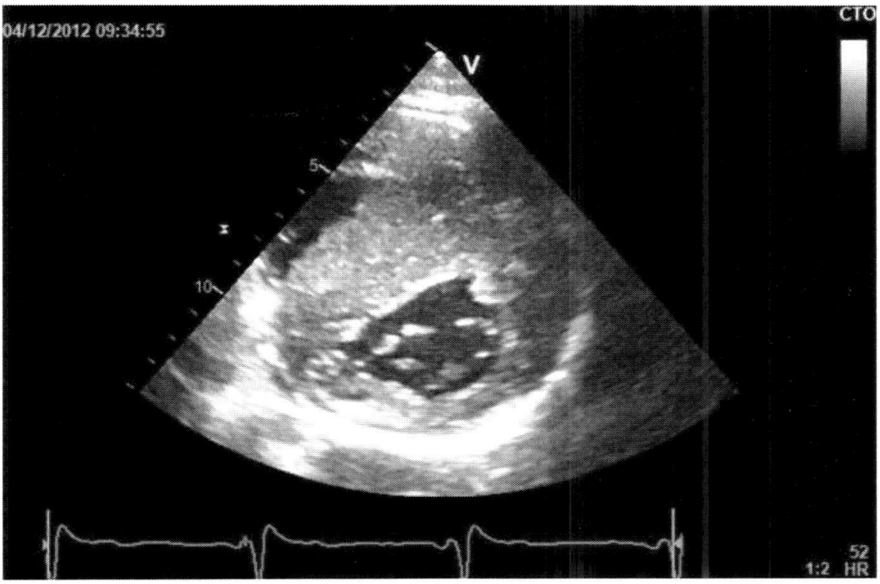

Figure 1. Parasternal short axis view demonstrating massive septal hypertrophy characterized by a septal diastolic thickness > 30 mm.

In a recent study (Vriesendorp et al. 2015), which was the first external and independent validation of the new model proposed by the recent guidelines (ESC guidelines) (Authors/Task Force members et al. 2014)), the left ventricular wall thickness and a thickness ≥30 mm were together the only predictors for SCD (Hazard ratio was 4.6, p= 0.003 for a thickness ≥30 mm).

Left Ventricular Ejection Fraction

Left ventricular ejection fraction is frequently normal or supernormal in Hypertrophic cardiomyopathy (HCM). However, a small number of

HCM patients progress to LV remodeling and systolic dysfunction (ejection fraction below 50%) referred to as end-stage HCM (B. J. Maron and Spirito 1998).

The reported prevalence of end-stage HCM varies from 2.4% to 15.7% in different series (Harris et al. 2006; Kawarai et al. 2011).

Some studies have pointed out that patients who develop a left ventricular dilatation have a high rate of complications and a lower rate of survival (Vassalli, Seiler, and Hess 1994).

Systolic function deterioration has been associated with increased mortality (up to 11% per year) and sudden cardiac death (Kawarai et al. 2011; Olivotto et al. 2012).

HCM is, effectively, not a static disease and Olivotto (Olivotto et al. 2012) identified 4 clinical stages of HCM including: nonhypertrophic HCM, classic phenotype, adverse remodeling and overt dysfunction (i.e., end stage phase).

Adverse remodeling (LVEF between 50% and 65% and increasing LV fibrosis) can occur in middle age, along with LV wall thickness regression (1–2 mm/yr), LV cavity enlargement (1–4 mm/yr) and decreased LVEF (B. J. Maron and Spirito 1998).

Over a period of approximately 5 to 6 years, the end-stage phase (LVEF <50% and extreme degrees of fibrosis) develops in 5% to 10% of patients with HCM.

Myocardial ischemia is a major pathophysiological mechanism of adverse remodeling in HCM (M. S. Maron et al. 2009).

As a result, myocardial cells die progressively (necrosis or apoptosis) and are replaced by fibrosis.

Olivotto (Olivotto et al. 2012) demonstrated that this progression is associated with an increase of SCD risk: from 0.5% to 1%/y in patients with classic phenotype to 10%/y in patients with LV overt dysfunction. This increase in risk was not considered in conventional risk prediction models.

According to ACCF/AHA guidelines, end-stage HCM is a class IIb indication for prophylactic ICD implantation in the absence of other risk factors for SCD (Gersh et al. 2011).

However, the new HCM Risk-SCD model is partially based on factors of disease progression including maximal left ventricular wall thickness, LA diameter, and left ventricular outflow tract gradient.

LEFT VENTRICLE OBSTRUCTION

Resting left ventricle obstruction (LVO) (gradient ≥30 mm Hg) is present in only one third of patients with HCM (Figure 2). Most patients with HCM do not exhibit significant resting LVO but a dynamic provoked gradient occurs in 25–30% of patients.

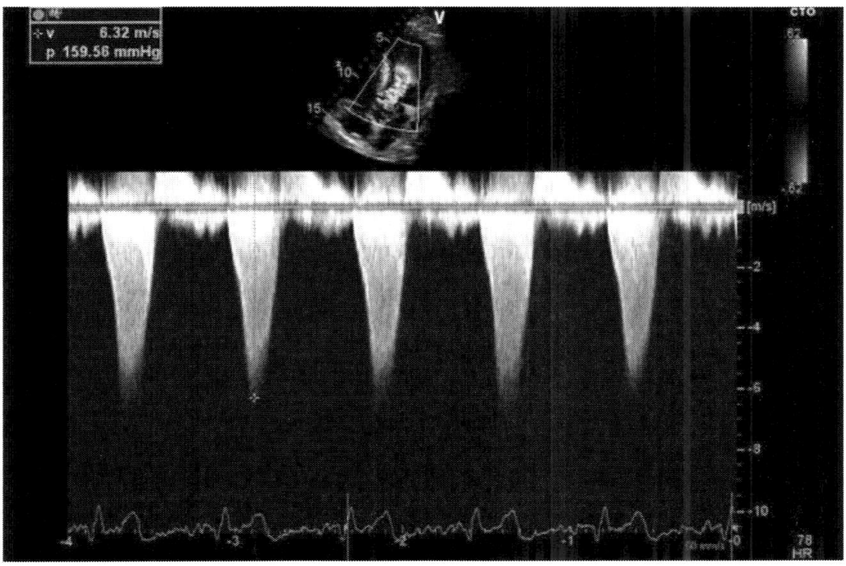

Figure 2. Left vernticular outflow tract obstruction with a high gradient (159 mmHg) in a patient with an asymmetric HCM.

Although some studies have not found a significant association between LVOT obstruction and SCD (Perry M. Elliott et al. 2006), other studies have found higher rates of SCD and progression to heart failure among patients with resting gradients ≥ 30 mm Hg (Barry J. Maron et al.

2009). This risk of SCD will be reduced after relief of obstruction by surgical myectomy (Dearani et al. 2007).

It was recently demonstrated that the proportion of HCM patients who develop NYHA functional class III/IV symptoms, as well as the rate of heart failure progression, is higher in patients with provocable or rest obstruction than among nonobstructive HCM patients (M. S. Maron et al. 2016).

LVO was considered an additional "risk modifier" and has been included in the 2011 ACCF/AHA guidelines on HCM.

Patients with nonobstructive cardiomyopathy (NOCM) are thought to be at relatively low risk compared to those with obstructive HCM.

This finding was not observed in the recent large study-level meta-analysis (Pelliccia et al. 2017) showing that annual mortality of patients with NOCM is not negligible and not significantly different from obstructive form (1.55% in non obstructive and 1.77% in obstructive form, $p=0.40$).

However, differences in the diagnostic criteria among studies was an important limitation and stress testing for assessing the obstruction was only used in a few studies.

Recently, Lu (Lu et al. 2017) proposed a novel HCM classification which divides LVOT gradients into four groups (rather than three); He distinguished two latent obstructive groups based on provoked gradient cut-offs at 30 and 90 mmHg.

- Patients with provoked gradients 30–89 mmHg who had the best prognosis, called "benign" latent obstructive HCM.
- Patients with provoked gradients ≥90 mmHg who had an intermediate risk for CV events, called "adverse" latent obstructive HCM.

The events included new onset atrial fibrillation, ventricular tachycardia/fibrillation, heart failure, transplantation, and death.

This new classification of obstruction can be seen in a new algorithm proposed by Lu (Figure 3).

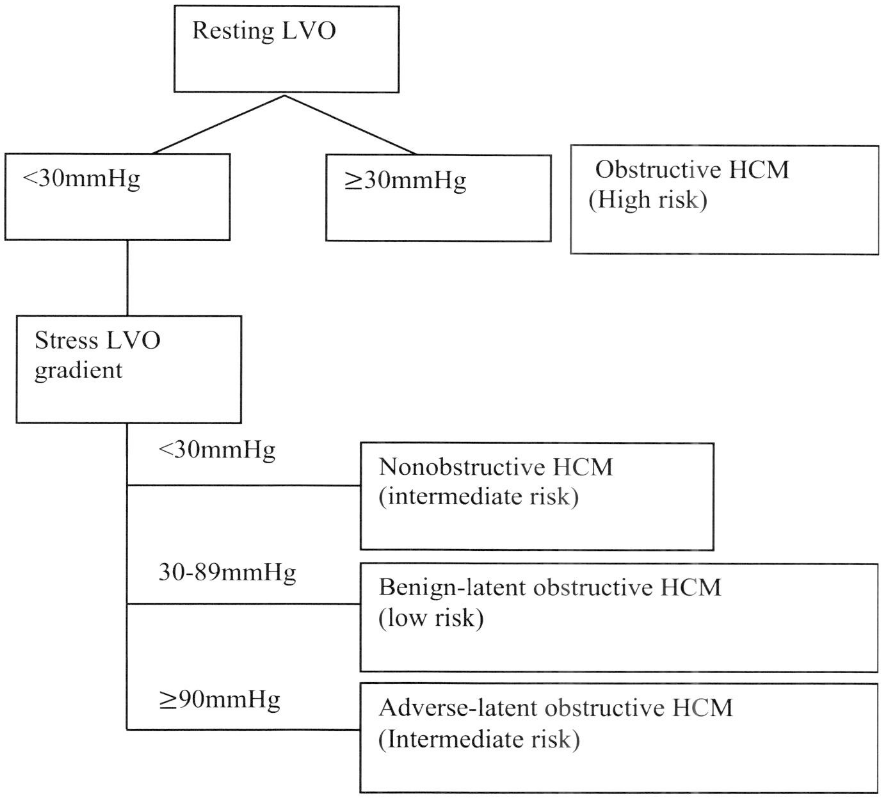

Figure 3. New proposed classification of obstruction in hypertrophic cardiomyopathy (Lu et al. 2017).

In this study, the nonobstructive HCM group, with low stress-induced LVOT gradients, was considered at intermediate risk.

This response to exercise may not always be benign and it was demonstrated in a previous study (Pozios et al. 2015), that non-obstructive hemodynamics is an independent predictor for ventricular tachycardia/fibrillation, and is associated with more extensive fibrosis and microvascular ischemia.

Therefore, in this study, obstructive HCM remains the subgroup with a clinical risk higher than all other sub-groups and may warrant more aggressive treatment strategies. At the same time, 30 mmHg is still seen as the most efficient threshold value for predicting adverse events.

The combination of rest and provoked gradients may help distinguish between low, intermediate and high-risk groups better.

The major finding is that patients with provoked gradients <30 mmHg or ≥90 mmHg are at an intermediate risk of adverse events, which is higher when compared to those with provoked gradients between 30 mmHg and 89 mmHg.

Recent studies found that those patients with a labile LV gradient had a better life expectancy than obstructive HCM and NOCM patients (M. S. Maron et al. 2016).

Left Ventricular Strain

Ejection fraction is usually preserved despite significant impairment of longitudinal contractile function, evidenced by attenuation in systolic annular velocities, strain and strain rate. With the use of strain imaging, it is now possible to identify regional heterogeneity in contractile function, an important advance in our understanding of myocardial mechanics in HCM.

In the terminal phase of the disease process, myocardial fibrosis may result in progressive impairment of systolic function in end-stage HCM.

2D strain makes spatial and temporal tracking of longitudinal, circumferential and radial myocardial deformation possible. Its ability to provide angle-independent measures of LV strain is advantageous.

Patients with HCM have significantly decreased longitudinal, circumferential, and radial strains compared to a healthy control group. Significant reductions in strain in the septal segments (particularly the mid-septal segment) correlate with the septal/posterior wall ratio.

Longitudinal strain analysis by 2D strain enables early detection of left ventricular contraction abnormalities in patients with HCM as well as preserved ejection fraction.

In addition, reduced global longitudinal strain (GLS) was found to be an independent factor associated with poor cardiac outcomes, particularly HF outcomes (Reant et al. 2016).

Abnormalities in myocardial mechanics are found at the site of abnormal myocardial hypertrophy (Yang et al. 2010).

Reant (Reant et al. 2015) demonstrated that lower GLS values correlate with several prognostic markers and reflect a more intrinsic myocyte dysfunction than other markers.

In this study, the type III pattern of Maron's classification (B. J. Maron, Gottdiener, and Epstein 1981) (septum and at least part of LV free wall) exhibits a worse profile than other patterns, with significantly lower GLS values.

Hiemstra (Hiemstra et al. 2017) recently demonstrated that GLS is independently associated with an adverse outcome in patients with HCM. Additionally, patients with GLS $\geq -15\%$ had a worse outcome compared to those with GLS $< -15\%$.

This cut-off value of −15% for GLS showed significant incremental value over clinical and standard echocardiographic parameters and may help optimize risk stratification.

The longitudinal strain probably reflects the characteristics of myocardial fiber disarray, myocardial fibrosis and microvascular dysfunction in patients with HCM (Saito et al. 2012).

This cut-off value for GLS was concordant with the value of -16% found in the recent study done by Liu (Liu et al. 2017) which demonstrated that event rates increased as GLS worsened.

This study also identified a high-risk group (those with GLS >-10%) who had significantly higher event rates compared with the other GLS subgroups.

There is no recommendation for preventing HF related to HCM and GLS seems to be of particular prognostic interest in this context. However, the best cut-off value to use in practice must be defined (Reant et al. 2016).

Recently, longer mechanical dispersion and decreased global longitudinal strain by speckle tracking echocardiography were found to be independent predictors of the occurrence of appropriate ICD therapy during the follow-up of sixty-three patients with hypertrophic cardiomyopathy (Candan et al. 2017).

Mechanical dispersion is defined as the standard deviation of time to peak negative strain in all left ventricular segments and reflects electrical abnormality and heterogeneity between these segments.

Echocardiographic Pattern of Principal Phenotypes

- Mid-ventricular hypertrophy

Hypertrophy is located only in the mid portion of the left ventricle and involves the papillary muscles, frequently resulting in systolic obstruction of the mid-ventricle (Parato et al. 2016).

As previously shown (Cai et al. 2014), midventricular obstructive HCM is more likely to develop systolic dysfunction, especially with apical aneurysms.

This finding was confirmed in Xiao's study (Xiao et al. 2015) which found that midventricular obstructive HCM was a main subtype of evolution into the end-stage phase.

LV mid-cavity obstruction is predominantly caused by marked septal hypertrophy coming in contact with a hypercontractile left ventricular free wall, often with the interposition of the hypertrophied papillary muscle. It occurs in approximately 10% of patients with HCM.

Some studies have shown an increased risk of SCD and progressive heart failure in these patients (Minami et al. 2011; Efthimiadis et al. 2013).

- LV apical aneurysm

LV apical aneurysm is defined as a discrete thin-walled dyskinetic or akinetic segment of the distal portion of the LV chamber with communication to the LV cavity (M. S. Maron et al. 2008). Echocardiography with contrast makes it possible to visualize these aneurysms better.

The incidence of apical aneurysm is approximately 1–2% of all HCM cases (Figure 4). It occurs in 25% of patients with LV mid-cavity obstruction and is also associated with higher cardiovascular events with an annual event rate of 10.5% per year including sudden death, appropriate ICD discharges, non-fatal thromboembolic stroke, progressive heart failure and death (M. S. Maron et al. 2008; Efthimiadis et al. 2013).

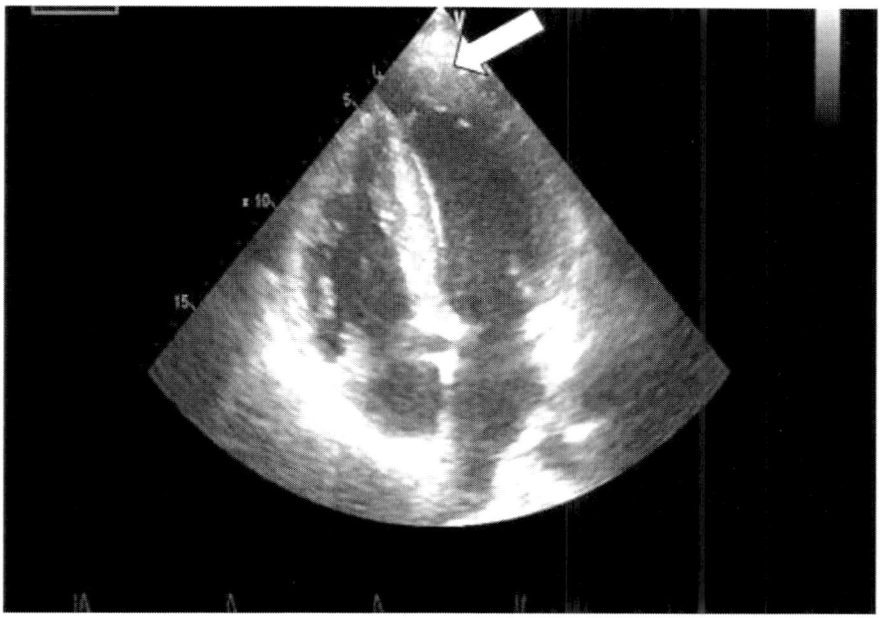

Figure 4. Left ventricular apical aneurysm in a patient with an asymmetric HCM and a high HCM-risk score.

Patients with a large apical aneurysm (>4 cm) were more likely to experience an adverse event.

It has been suggested that LV apical aneurysm can be used to guide ICD therapy in individuals who are at intermediate risk, but there is little data to support this approach (M. S. Maron et al. 2008).

In the recent ESC risk score, this parameter was not included.

This was recently assessed further on a large group of patients (1940 patients) over an extended period of time (Rowin et al. 2017).

Left ventricular apical aneurysm was identified in 93 patients (4.8%).

Combining mortality and nonfatal adverse HCM-related events, apical aneurysm patients had a 3-fold greater event rate than the 1,847 patients without aneurysms (6.4%/year vs. 2.0%/year; $p < 0.001$), as well as a 5-fold higher rate of arrhythmic events (4.7%/year vs. 0.9%/year; $p < 0.001$).

Otherwise, there was no consistent relationship between aneurysm size and outcome endpoints.

In this study, only 2 (10%) of the 21 LV aneurysm patients with arrhythmic events, were judged to be at high risk based on the recent ESC risk score (>6%/5 years). Thirteen of the 21 patients (62%) were judged to be at low risk (<4%/5 years), considered insufficient to recommend an ICD.

- Apical and Asymmetric Septal Hypertrophic Cardiomyopathy

An (An et al. 2017) compared the long-term outcome between apical hypertrophic cardiomyopathy (ApHCM) and asymmetric septal hypertrophic cardiomyopathy (ASHCM) in 540 patients.

After eliminating the interference of diagnostic age, gender and outflow tract obstruction, ASHCM had a worse prognosis with a higher incidence of cardiovascular mortality and morbidity than ApHCM.

The favorable outcome of apical HCM, when compared with other forms of HCM, was confirmed in Kim's study (Kim et al. 2016).

Conclusion

Behind its diagnostic value, echocardiography is also a tool for the prognostic assessment of HCM.

Several echocardiographic parameters are important for predicting unfavorable outcome in HCM patients including maximal wall thickness >30mm, LVOT gradient at rest >30mmHg, EF <50%, and left atrial dimension.

The echocardiographic pattern of the different phenotypes significantly impacts the prognosis of this disease.

Recent strain parameters are promising to stratify risk in HCM but need more study to be included in the scores of SCD.

References

An, Shuoyan, Chaomei Fan, Lirong Yan, Chi Cai, Yinjian Yang, Shanshan Zhai, Shihua Zhao, et al. 2017. "Comparison of Long-Term Outcome between Apical and Asymmetric Septal Hypertrophic Cardiomyopathy." *Cardiology* 136 (2): 108–14. doi:10.1159/000448239.

Authors/Task Force members, Perry M. Elliott, Aris Anastasakis, Michael A. Borger, Martin Borggrefe, Franco Cecchi, Philippe Charron, et al. 2014. "2014 ESC Guidelines on Diagnosis and Management of Hypertrophic Cardiomyopathy: The Task Force for the Diagnosis and Management of Hypertrophic Cardiomyopathy of the European Society of Cardiology (ESC)." *European Heart Journal* 35 (39): 2733–79. doi:10.1093/eurheartj/ehu284.

Cai, Chi, Fu-jian Duan, Yin-jian Yang, Xi-ying Guo, Yan-ling Liu, Yu-qing Liu, Li-rong Yan, et al. 2014. "Comparison of the Prevalence, Clinical Features, and Long-Term Outcomes of Midventricular Hypertrophy vs Apical Phenotype in Patients with Hypertrophic Cardiomyopathy." *The Canadian Journal of Cardiology* 30 (4): 441–47. doi:10.1016/j.cjca.2013.10.005.

Candan, Ozkan, Cetin Gecmen, Emrah Bayam, Ahmet Guner, Mehmet Celik, and Cem Doğan. 2017. "Mechanical Dispersion and Global Longitudinal Strain by Speckle Tracking Echocardiography: Predictors of Appropriate Implantable Cardioverter Defibrillator Therapy in Hypertrophic Cardiomyopathy." *Echocardiography (Mount Kisco, N.Y.)* 34 (6): 835–42. doi:10.1111/echo.13547.

Dearani, Joseph A., Steve R. Ommen, Bernard J. Gersh, Hartzell V. Schaff, and Gordon K. Danielson. 2007. "Surgery Insight: Septal

Myectomy for Obstructive Hypertrophic Cardiomyopathy--the Mayo Clinic Experience." *Nature Clinical Practice. Cardiovascular Medicine* 4 (9): 503–12. doi:10.1038/ncpcardio0965.

Debonnaire, Philippe, Emer Joyce, Yasmine Hiemstra, Bart J. Mertens, Douwe E. Atsma, Martin J. Schalij, Jeroen J. Bax, Victoria Delgado, and Nina Ajmone Marsan. 2017. "Left Atrial Size and Function in Hypertrophic Cardiomyopathy Patients and Risk of New-Onset Atrial Fibrillation." *Circulation. Arrhythmia and Electrophysiology* 10 (2). doi:10.1161/CIRCEP.116.004052.

Dimitrow, Pawel Petkow, Lidia Chojnowska, Tomasz Rudzinski, Walerian Piotrowski, Lidia Ziólkowska, Andrzej Wojtarowicz, Anna Wycisk, et al. 2010. "Sudden Death in Hypertrophic Cardiomyopathy: Old Risk Factors Re-Assessed in a New Model of Maximalized Follow-Up." *European Heart Journal* 31 (24): 3084–93. doi:10.1093/eurheartj/ehq308.

Efthimiadis, Georgios K., Efstathios D. Pagourelias, Despoina Parcharidou, Thomas Gossios, Vasileios Kamperidis, Efstratios K. Theofilogiannakos, Zoi Pappa, et al. 2013. "Clinical Characteristics and Natural History of Hypertrophic Cardiomyopathy with Midventricular Obstruction." *Circulation Journal: Official Journal of the Japanese Circulation Society* 77 (9): 2366–74.

Elliott, P. M., J. R. Gimeno Blanes, N. G. Mahon, J. D. Poloniecki, and W. J. McKenna. 2001. "Relation between Severity of Left-Ventricular Hypertrophy and Prognosis in Patients with Hypertrophic Cardiomyopathy." *Lancet (London, England)* 357 (9254): 420–24. doi:10.1016/S0140-6736(00)04005-8.

Elliott, Perry M., Juan R. Gimeno, María T. Tomé, Jaymin Shah, Deirdre Ward, Rajesh Thaman, Jens Mogensen, and William J. McKenna. 2006. "Left Ventricular Outflow Tract Obstruction and Sudden Death Risk in Patients with Hypertrophic Cardiomyopathy." *European Heart Journal* 27 (16): 1933–41. doi:10.1093/eurheartj/ehl041.

Gersh, Bernard J., Barry J. Maron, Robert O. Bonow, Joseph A. Dearani, Michael A. Fifer, Mark S. Link, Srihari S. Naidu, et al. 2011. "2011 ACCF/AHA Guideline for the Diagnosis and Treatment of

Hypertrophic Cardiomyopathy: A Report of the American College of Cardiology Foundation/American Heart Association Task Force on Practice Guidelines Developed in Collaboration With the American Association for Thoracic Surgery, American Society of Echocardiography, American Society of Nuclear Cardiology, Heart Failure Society of America, Heart Rhythm Society, Society for Cardiovascular Angiography and Interventions, and Society of Thoracic Surgeons." *Journal of the American College of Cardiology* 58 (25): e212–60. doi:10.1016/j.jacc.2011.06.011.

Harris, Kevin M., Paolo Spirito, Martin S. Maron, Andrey G. Zenovich, Francesco Formisano, John R. Lesser, Shannon Mackey-Bojack, Warren J. Manning, James E. Udelson, and Barry J. Maron. 2006. "Prevalence, Clinical Profile, and Significance of Left Ventricular Remodeling in the End-Stage Phase of Hypertrophic Cardiomyopathy." *Circulation* 114 (3): 216–25. doi:10.1161/CIRCULATIONAHA.105.583500.

Hiemstra, Yasmine L., Philippe Debonnaire, Marianne Bootsma, Erik W. van Zwet, Victoria Delgado, Martin J. Schalij, Douwe E. Atsma, Jeroen J. Bax, and Nina Ajmone Marsan. 2017. "Global Longitudinal Strain and Left Atrial Volume Index Provide Incremental Prognostic Value in Patients With Hypertrophic Cardiomyopathy." *Circulation. Cardiovascular Imaging* 10 (7). doi:10.1161/CIRCIMAGING.116.005706.

Kawarai, Hirotaka, Katsuya Kajimoto, Yuichiro Minami, Nobuhisa Hagiwara, and Hiroshi Kasanuki. 2011. "Risk of Sudden Death in End-Stage Hypertrophic Cardiomyopathy." *Journal of Cardiac Failure* 17 (6): 459–64. doi:10.1016/j.cardfail.2011.01.015.

Kim, Eun Kyoung, Sang-Chol Lee, Ji Won Hwang, Sung-A. Chang, Sung-Ji Park, Young Keun On, Kyoung Min Park, et al. 2016. "Differences in Apical and Non-Apical Types of Hypertrophic Cardiomyopathy: A Prospective Analysis of Clinical, Echocardiographic, and Cardiac Magnetic Resonance Findings and Outcome from 350 Patients." *European Heart Journal Cardiovascular Imaging* 17 (6): 678–86. doi:10.1093/ehjci/jev192.

Lang, Roberto M., Luigi P. Badano, Victor Mor-Avi, Jonathan Afilalo, Anderson Armstrong, Laura Ernande, Frank A. Flachskampf, et al. 2015. "Recommendations for Cardiac Chamber Quantification by Echocardiography in Adults: An Update from the American Society of Echocardiography and the European Association of Cardiovascular Imaging." *Journal of the American Society of Echocardiography: Official Publication of the American Society of Echocardiography* 28 (1): 1–39.e14. doi:10.1016/j.echo.2014.10.003.

Liu, Hongyun, Iraklis Pozios, Bereketeab Haileselassie, Alexandra Nowbar, Lars L. Sorensen, Susan Phillip, Dai-Yin Lu, et al. 2017. "Role of Global Longitudinal Strain in Predicting Outcomes in Hypertrophic Cardiomyopathy." *The American Journal of Cardiology* 120 (4): 670–75. doi:10.1016/j.amjcard.2017.05.039.

Losi, Maria-Angela, Sandro Betocchi, Giovanni Barbati, Valentina Parisi, Carlo-Gabriele Tocchetti, Fabio Pastore, Teresa Migliore, et al. 2009. "Prognostic Significance of Left Atrial Volume Dilatation in Patients with Hypertrophic Cardiomyopathy." *Journal of the American Society of Echocardiography: Official Publication of the American Society of Echocardiography* 22 (1): 76–81. doi:10.1016/j.echo.2008.11.001.

Louie, E. K., and B. J. Maron. 1986. "Hypertrophic Cardiomyopathy with Extreme Increase in Left Ventricular Wall Thickness: Functional and Morphologic Features and Clinical Significance." *Journal of the American College of Cardiology* 8 (1): 57–65.

Lu, Dai-Yin, Bereketeab Hailesealassie, Ioannis Ventoulis, Hongyun Liu, Hsin-Yueh Liang, Alexandra Nowbar, Iraklis Pozios, et al. 2017. "Impact of Peak Provoked Left Ventricular Outflow Tract Gradients on Clinical Outcomes in Hypertrophic Cardiomyopathy." *International Journal of Cardiology* 243 (September): 290–95. doi:10.1016/j.ijcard. 2017.04.039.

Marian, Ali J. 2010. "Hypertrophic Cardiomyopathy: From Genetics to Treatment." *European Journal of Clinical Investigation* 40 (4): 360–69.

Maron, B. J., J. S. Gottdiener, and S. E. Epstein. 1981. "Patterns and Significance of Distribution of Left Ventricular Hypertrophy in

Hypertrophic Cardiomyopathy. A Wide Angle, Two Dimensional Echocardiographic Study of 125 Patients." *The American Journal of Cardiology* 48 (3): 418–28.

Maron, B. J., and P. Spirito. 1998. "Implications of Left Ventricular Remodeling in Hypertrophic Cardiomyopathy." *The American Journal of Cardiology* 81 (11): 1339–44.

Maron, Barry J., Martin S. Maron, E. Douglas Wigle, and Eugene Braunwald. 2009. "The 50-Year History, Controversy, and Clinical Implications of Left Ventricular Outflow Tract Obstruction in Hypertrophic Cardiomyopathy from Idiopathic Hypertrophic Subaortic Stenosis to Hypertrophic Cardiomyopathy: From Idiopathic Hypertrophic Subaortic Stenosis to Hypertrophic Cardiomyopathy." *Journal of the American College of Cardiology* 54 (3): 191–200. doi:10.1016/j.jacc.2008.11.069.

Maron, Martin S., John J. Finley, J. Martijn Bos, Thomas H. Hauser, Warren J. Manning, Tammy S. Haas, John R. Lesser, James E. Udelson, Michael J. Ackerman, and Barry J. Maron. 2008. "Prevalence, Clinical Significance, and Natural History of Left Ventricular Apical Aneurysms in Hypertrophic Cardiomyopathy." *Circulation* 118 (15): 1541–49. doi:10.1161/CIRCULATIONAHA. 108.781401.

Maron, Martin S., Iacopo Olivotto, Barry J. Maron, Sanjay K. Prasad, Franco Cecchi, James E. Udelson, and Paolo G. Camici. 2009. "The Case for Myocardial Ischemia in Hypertrophic Cardiomyopathy." *Journal of the American College of Cardiology* 54 (9): 866–75. doi:10.1016/j.jacc.2009.04.072.

Maron, Martin S., Ethan J. Rowin, Iacopo Olivotto, Susan A. Casey, Anna Arretini, Benedetta Tomberli, Ross F. Garberich, et al. 2016. "Contemporary Natural History and Management of Nonobstructive Hypertrophic Cardiomyopathy." *Journal of the American College of Cardiology* 67 (12): 1399–1409. doi:10.1016/j.jacc.2016.01.023.

Minami, Yuichiro, Katsuya Kajimoto, Yutaka Terajima, Bun Yashiro, Dai Okayama, Shintaro Haruki, Takatomo Nakajima, Naomi Kawashiro, Masatoshi Kawana, and Nobuhisa Hagiwara. 2011. "Clinical

Implications of Midventricular Obstruction in Patients with Hypertrophic Cardiomyopathy." *Journal of the American College of Cardiology* 57 (23): 2346–55. doi:10.1016/j.jacc.2011.02.033.

Olivotto, Iacopo, Franco Cecchi, Corrado Poggesi, and Magdi H. Yacoub. 2012. "Patterns of Disease Progression in Hypertrophic Cardiomyopathy: An Individualized Approach to Clinical Staging." *Circulation. Heart Failure* 5 (4): 535–46. doi:10.1161/CIRCHEART FAILURE.112.967026.

O'Mahony, Constantinos, Fatima Jichi, Menelaos Pavlou, Lorenzo Monserrat, Aristides Anastasakis, Claudio Rapezzi, Elena Biagini, et al. 2014. "A Novel Clinical Risk Prediction Model for Sudden Cardiac Death in Hypertrophic Cardiomyopathy (HCM Risk-SCD)." *European Heart Journal* 35 (30): 2010–20. doi:10.1093/eurheartj/eht439.

Parato, Vito Maurizio, Valeria Antoncecchi, Fabiola Sozzi, Stefania Marazia, Annapaola Zito, Maria Maiello, Pasquale Palmiero, and Italian Chapter of ISCU. 2016. "Echocardiographic Diagnosis of the Different Phenotypes of Hypertrophic Cardiomyopathy." *Cardiovascular Ultrasound* 14 (1):30.doi:10.1186/s12947-016-0072-5.

Pelliccia, Francesco, Vincenzo Pasceri, Giuseppe Limongelli, Camillo Autore, Cristina Basso, Domenico Corrado, Massimo Imazio, et al. 2017. "Long-Term Outcome of Nonobstructive versus Obstructive Hypertrophic Cardiomyopathy: A Systematic Review and Meta-Analysis." *International Journal of Cardiology* 243 (September): 379–84. doi:10.1016/j.ijcard.2017.06.071.

Pozios, Iraklis, Celia Corona-Villalobos, Lars L. Sorensen, Paco E. Bravo, Marco Canepa, Chiara Pisanello, Aurelio Pinheiro, et al. 2015. "Comparison of Outcomes in Patients With Nonobstructive, Labile-Obstructive, and Chronically Obstructive Hypertrophic Cardiomyopathy." *The American Journal of Cardiology* 116 (6): 938–44. doi:10.1016/j.amjcard.2015.06.018.

Reant, Patricia, Erwan Donal, Frederic Schnell, Amelie Reynaud, Magalie Daudin, Xavier Pillois, Marina Dijos, et al. 2015. "Clinical and Imaging Description of the Maron Subtypes of Hypertrophic

Cardiomyopathy." *The International Journal of Cardiovascular Imaging* 31 (1): 47–55. doi:10.1007/s10554-014-0529-2.

Reant, Patricia, Mariana Mirabel, Guy Lloyd, Jérôme Peyrou, Jose-Maria Lopez Ayala, Shaughan Dickie, Heeraj Bulluck, et al. 2016. "Global Longitudinal Strain Is Associated with Heart Failure Outcomes in Hypertrophic Cardiomyopathy." *Heart (British Cardiac Society)* 102 (10): 741–47. doi:10.1136/heartjnl-2015-308576.

Rowin, Ethan J., Barry J. Maron, Tammy S. Haas, Ross F. Garberich, Weijia Wang, Mark S. Link, and Martin S. Maron. 2017. "Hypertrophic Cardiomyopathy With Left Ventricular Apical Aneurysm: Implications for Risk Stratification and Management." *Journal of the American College of Cardiology* 69 (7): 761–73. doi:10.1016/j.jacc.2016.11.063.

Saito, Makoto, Hideki Okayama, Toyofumi Yoshii, Haruhiko Higashi, Hiroe Morioka, Go Hiasa, Takumi Sumimoto, et al. 2012. "Clinical Significance of Global Two-Dimensional Strain as a Surrogate Parameter of Myocardial Fibrosis and Cardiac Events in Patients with Hypertrophic Cardiomyopathy." *European Heart Journal Cardiovascular Imaging* 13 (7): 617–23. doi:10.1093/ejechocard/jer318.

Sorajja, Paul, Rick A. Nishimura, Steve R. Ommen, Michael J. Ackerman, A. Jamil Tajik, and Bernard J. Gersh. 2006. "Use of Echocardiography in Patients with Hypertrophic Cardiomyopathy: Clinical Implications of Massive Hypertrophy." *Journal of the American Society of Echocardiography: Official Publication of the American Society of Echocardiography* 19 (6): 788–95. doi:10.1016/j.echo.2006.01.005.

Spirito, P., P. Bellone, K. M. Harris, P. Bernabo, P. Bruzzi, and B. J. Maron. 2000. "Magnitude of Left Ventricular Hypertrophy and Risk of Sudden Death in Hypertrophic Cardiomyopathy." *The New England Journal of Medicine* 342 (24): 1778–85. doi:10.1056/NEJM200006153422403.

Spirito, P., and B. J. Maron. 1987. "Absence of Progression of Left Ventricular Hypertrophy in Adult Patients with Hypertrophic

Cardiomyopathy." *Journal of the American College of Cardiology* 9 (5): 1013–17.

Spirito, Paolo, Camillo Autore, Claudio Rapezzi, Paola Bernabò, Roberto Badagliacca, Martin S. Maron, Sergio Bongioanni, et al. 2009. "Syncope and Risk of Sudden Death in Hypertrophic Cardiomyopathy." *Circulation* 119 (13): 1703–10. doi:10.1161/CIRCULATIONAHA.108.798314.

Vassalli, G., C. Seiler, and O. M. Hess. 1994. "Risk Stratification in Hypertrophic Cardiomyopathy." *Current Opinion in Cardiology* 9 (3): 330–36.

Vriesendorp, Pieter A., Arend F. L. Schinkel, Max Liebregts, Dominic A. M. J. Theuns, Johan van Cleemput, Folkert J. Ten Cate, Rik Willems, and Michelle Michels. 2015. "Validation of the 2014 European Society of Cardiology Guidelines Risk Prediction Model for the Primary Prevention of Sudden Cardiac Death in Hypertrophic Cardiomyopathy." *Circulation. Arrhythmia and Electrophysiology* 8 (4): 829–35. doi:10.1161/CIRCEP.114.002553.

Xiao, Yan, Kun-Qi Yang, Yan-Kun Yang, Ya-Xin Liu, Tao Tian, Lei Song, Xiong-Jing Jiang, and Xian-Liang Zhou. 2015. "Clinical Characteristics and Prognosis of End-Stage Hypertrophic Cardiomyopathy." *Chinese Medical Journal* 128 (11): 1483–89. doi:10.4103/0366-6999.157656.

Yang, Hua, Shemy Carasso, Anna Woo, Michal Jamorski, Anna Nikonova, E. Douglas Wigle, and Harry Rakowski. 2010. "Hypertrophy Pattern and Regional Myocardial Mechanics Are Related in Septal and Apical Hypertrophic Cardiomyopathy." *Journal of the American Society of Echocardiography: Official Publication of the American Society of Echocardiography* 23 (10): 1081–89. doi:10.1016/j.echo.2010.06.006.

In: Hypertrophic Cardiomyopathy
Editor: Ikram Kammoun
ISBN: 978-1-53613-003-4

Chapter 6

Risk Stratification of Sudden Cardiac Death in Hypertrophic Cardiomyopathy

Sonia Marrakchi[1,*], MD, Ikram Kammoun[1], Emna Bennour[1], Françoise Hidden Lucet[2] and Salem Kachboura[1]

[1]Department of cardiology, Tunis ElManar University, Ariana, Tunisia
[2]Department of cardiology, Pitie-Salpetriere Hospital – APHP, Paris, France

Abstract

Sudden cardiac death (SCD) is the most devastating complication of hypertrophic cardiomyopathy (HCM). The greatest challenge in the management of HCM is identifying those at increased risk as an implantable cardioverter defibrillator (ICD) is a potentially life-saving therapy.

We sought to summarize the available data on SCD in HCM and provide a clinical perspective on the current differing and somewhat conflicting data on risk stratification. Additionally, we sought to learn

* Corresponding author: marrakchi.sonia@yahoo.fr.

more about the actual implementation of guidelines by HCM experts worldwide.

The HCM Risk-SCD model improves risk stratification of HCM patients for primary prevention of SCD, and calculating an individual risk estimate contributes to the clinical decision-making process. Improved risk stratification is important for decision-making before ICD implantation for primary prevention of SCD.

Keywords: hypertrophic cardiomyopathy, risk prediction, sudden cardiac death

INTRODUCTION

Hypertrophic cardiomyopathy (HCM) is the most common form of genetically inherited cardiovascular disease, with a prevalence of one in 500 individuals (Barry J. Maron et al. 2014; B. J. Maron et al. 1995). HCM, a genetic sarcomeric disorder responsible for myocyte and myofibrillar disarray and interstitial fibrosis, is intimately linked to sudden cardiac death (SCD) due to malignant ventricular arrhythmias (Trivedi and Knight 2016).

Mortality rates in early studies were as high as 5–7% per year (Hardarson et al. 1973). With the advent of the implantable cardioverter defibrillator (ICD) and early detection of the disease, modern cohorts have mortality rates of under 1% (B. J. Maron et al. 2000). SCD due to sustained ventricular tachycardia (VT) or ventricular fibrillation (VF) is still the most common cause of mortality, however, accounting for 51% of all HCM-related deaths (B. J. Maron et al. 2000). Sudden death in patients with HCM is one of the leading causes of death in individuals under the age of 40 (van der Werf, van Langen, and Wilde 2010).

In this article, we sought to summarize the available data on SCD in HCM and provide a clinical perspective on the current differing on risk stratification, with balanced guidance with regards to rational clinical decision-making. Additionally, we sought to learn more about the actual implementation of current guidelines by HCM experts worldwide (Weissler-Snir et al. 2017).

SUDDEN DEATH

Since the initial descriptions of HCM, sudden death has been a highly visible and devastating consequence of the disease (Rowin and Maron 2016). Fortunately, sudden death is confined to a small subset of patients with HCM within the broad disease spectrum (B. J. Maron et al. 2000; Rowin and Maron 2016). Sudden death events occur unpredictably, often without warning signs or symptoms and is most common in young to middle-aged people (Barry J. Maron et al. 2014).

The true prevalence of SCD in HCM is difficult to estimate, as a substantial portion of cases remain unrecognized (Weissler-Snir et al. 2017). Although the annual rate of SCD in the general HCM population is <1% per year according to contemporary series, there is still a small subset of patients who are at increased risk of SCD (B. J. Maron et al. 2000; Barry J. Maron, Rowin, et al. 2015). The application of ICD for primary prevention of sudden death in HCM has created the opportunity to prevent these catastrophic events (Barry J. Maron et al. 2007). This has placed increased importance on risk stratification to help identify individuals who may benefit from device therapy for primary prevention (Rowin and Maron 2016). The greatest challenge in the management of HCM is identifying those at increased risk, as an implantable cardioverter defibrillator (ICD) is a potentially life-saving therapy.

The current American College of Cardiology (ACC) and American Heart Association (AHA)-based HCM risk stratification algorithm has relied on five major risk markers and has been highly effective in identifying many patients with HCM who will benefit from ICD therapy (Gersh et al. 2011). While this has been instrumental in decreasing rates of sudden death and HCM-related mortality to 0.5% per year, some patients without conventional risk markers nevertheless remain at risk of sudden death (Barry J. Maron, Rowin, et al. 2015; B. J. Maron et al. 2000). These limitations have led to an interest in additional strategies to improve the current risk model.

ELECTROPHYSIOLOGY SUBSTRATUM

Hypertrophic cardiomyopathy is an inheritable myocardial disorder characterized by both increased ventricular wall thickness in the absence of other causative conditions and potentially fatal arrhythmias.

Autopsy observations have demonstrated a range of histopathological features which can be grouped into three distinct features, namely extensive disarray of hypertrophy myocytes and myofibrils, abnormalities of the intramural microvasculature, and increased interstitial and/or focal fibrosis (Weissler-Snir et al. 2017). This condition is a slowly progressive disorder that manifests remarkably variable clinical courses from near-normal life expectancy with no symptoms to sudden cardiac death (SCD) in youth (Kawashiri et al. 2014; Konno et al. 2003, 2010).

Under disease, adverse remodeling and cardiac fibrosis can become a persistent process, resulting in distorted cardiac architecture and function. This leads to mechanical stiffness and diastolic dysfunction and supports the development of cardiac arrhythmias (Disertori, Masè, and Ravelli 2017) by re-entrant ventricular arrhythmias (Varnava et al. 2001). Silent low-grade myocardial ischemia and altered coronary blood flow are common in HCM and help create the conditions needed for scar formation and arrhythmogenesis (Basso et al. 2000). Fibrosed and disrupted cellular architecture is often found throughout the heart, but is mostly concentrated in the densest area of hypertrophy (Chan et al. 2014a). Fibrosis and myofibroblast activation can favor the onset and maintenance of cardiac arrhythmias by different mechanisms. Increased collagen deposition with fibrosis results in myocyte electrical decoupling, affecting both conduction and impulse formation (Nguyen, Qu, and Weiss 2014; Morita et al. 2014). The degree of arrhythmogenicity depends on the amount of fibrosis, with maximal arrhythmia propensity occurring for intermediate levels of fibrosis (Morita et al. 2014), but also based on the texture of fibrosis. Compact fibrosis with large areas completely deprived by myocytes can favor arrhythmias by anchoring reentrant waves. Heterogeneous fibrosis with diffuse and patchy/interstitial forms play the major arrhythmogenic role (de Jong et al. 2011). The presence of non-conducting collagen septa between myocytes leads to conduction slowing and augmented anisotropy, and promotes the escape of ectopic beats, such as after depolarization-induced premature beats, and the formation of unidirectional conduction block by reducing source-sink mismatch (Nguyen, Qu, and Weiss 2014; Morita et al. 2014).

RISK STRATIFICATION

Although the current mortality rate of HCM is low, there are groups of patients with an elevated risk of SCD who would benefit from ICD placement. Estimating SCD risk is an integral part of clinical management. A large body of evidence suggests that, in adolescents and adults, risk assessment should include clinical and family history, 48-hour ambulatory ECG, TTE (or CMR in the case of poor echo windows) and a symptom-limited exercise test. Clinical features are associated with increased SCD risk and have been used in previous guidelines to estimate risk (Authors/Task Force members et al. 2014). The guidelines recommend that all patients should undergo SCD risk stratification at their initial evaluation, as well as periodic re-evaluation to determine whether their risk of SCD has changed (Gersh et al. 2011).

Originally, in the 2003 ACC/ESC guidelines and 2011 ACCF/AHA guidelines, the identification of high-risk patients was based on five characteristic parameters: a family history of SCD in first-degree relatives < 40 years of age, maximal left ventricular wall thickness (LVWT) >30 mm, unexplainable syncope, non-sustained ventricular tachycardia (NSVT) and abnormal blood pressure response during exercise (Barry J. Maron et al. 2003; Gersh et al. 2011). It was clear, however, that the risk of SCD increases with increasing number of risk factors. In the 2003 guidelines, each risk factor was of equal weight and the profile was calculated as the sum of all risk factors present in the patient. The approach for the 2011 guideline was similar, except that documented NSVT and abnormal blood pressure response during exercise are only considered if at least one of the other risk factors is present. The clinical variables are grouped into two categories. The first category includes established risk markers. Some of these markers are individually sufficient to prompt ICD placement. The second category includes risk modifiers. These serve as additional markers to help identify high-risk patients; alone they are not sufficient to recommend ICD placement (Gersh et al. 2011). The 2014 European guidelines also include left atrial diameter and LV outflow tract gradient as part of a risk-prediction scoring system which was not only validated in a multicenter, retrospective, longitudinal cohort study but was made into an online risk-prediction calculator which could theoretically improve the relative accuracy with which appropriateness of primary prevention ICDs could be evaluated (Betensky and Dixit 2014; Veselka, Anavekar, and Charron 2017). Identifying patients within this heterogeneous disorder who are at high risk of sudden death remains a challenge.

Major Clinical Features Associated with an Increased Risk of Sudden Cardiac Death in Adults

Risk factors most commonly cited include nonsustained VT, LV wall thickness >30mm, family history of SCD, unexplained syncope, and abnormal blood pressure response to exercise (Betensky and Dixit 2014). Other risk markers help identify high-risk patients like late gadolinium enhancement (LGE) on cardiac magnetic resonance imaging (cMRI), genetic mutations, LV apical aneurysms and systolic dysfunction (Gersh et al. 2011). The European guidelines also include: age, left atrial diameter and LV outflow tract gradient as part of a risk-prediction scoring system (Veselka, Anavekar, and Charron 2017).

Echocardiographic parameters including LV wall thickness, LV apical aneurysms, LV obstruction, LV systolic dysfunction and left atrial diameter were detailed in chapter six.

Prior Personal History of Ventricular Fibrillation, Sudden Cardiac Death or Sustained Ventricular Tachycardia

Patients who have already experienced and survived an episode of SCD or malignant ventricular arrhythmia represent the highest risk group. The annual rate of subsequent events in this secondary prevention group is 10% per year (Barry J. Maron et al. 2009; P. M. Elliott et al. 1999, 2000). This is the only risk marker with an excellent positive predictive value. Maron (Barry J. Maron et al. 2007) found that of 506 study patients, 123 (24%) received ICDs after a resuscitated cardiac arrest or sustained ventricular tachycardia. Of these 123 patients, 52 (42%) experienced appropriate ICD discharges. Intervention rate was 10.6% per year and cumulative probability of discharge after 5 years was 39%.

However, even this group of particularly high-risk patients may experience either no further recurrence or prolonged event-free intervals between arrhythmic episodes (Barry J. Maron et al. 2009; P. M. Elliott et al. 1999).

Age

Sudden death in patients with HCM is one of the leading causes of death in individuals under the age of 40 (van der Werf, van Langen, and Wilde 2010). While there appears to be no difference in SCD rates based on gender, age is an important factor (Iacopo Olivotto et al. 2005). SCD is more common in younger patients, especially those under the age of 35. Initial reports showed that SCD occurred almost exclusively in patients younger than 35 years of age (B. J. Maron, Roberts, and Epstein 1982).

Nonetheless, an international, multi-center study on 744 largely unselected patients with HCM has found that although SCD is more common among younger patients it is not confined to this group of patients and continued to occur throughout life. Up to 20% of SCDs have been reported to occur in patients over the age of 65 (B. J. Maron et al. 2000). However, a recent study on 428 HCM patients ≥60 years of age found that the risk of SCD in those patients was high and that chances of surviving into the seventh decade of life was low, even in the presence of conventional risk factors (Barry J. Maron et al. 2013).

This parameter was recently included in risk score (see below) in the new guidelines (Authors/Task Force members et al. 2014).

Non-Sustained Ventricular Tachycardia

NSVT is defined as ≥3 consecutive ventricular beats at ≥120 BPM lasting <30 seconds. It occurs in 20–30% of patients during ambulatory ECG monitoring and is an independent predictor of SCD (Monserrat et al. 2003; Gimeno et al. 2009; Dimitrow et al. 2010).

In previous studies, assessing the risk of SD in HCM, NSVT were commonly slow and short-lasting (Monserrat et al. 2003; Adabag et al. 2005; P. Spirito et al. 1994; Borggrefe et al. 1983).

However, short-lasting and relatively slow bursts of NSVT detected with Holter was not relates to SD in any tertiary cohorts (Adabag et al. 2005). Spirito (P. Spirito et al. 1994) showed in a 151-patient study that cardiac mortality is low in patients with hypertrophic cardiomyopathy who are asymptomatic or only mildly symptomatic and have brief and infrequent episodes of VT on ambulatory ECG monitoring.

Albeit never proven, it has been suggested that NSVT in HCM should not be considered in a simply binary manner, and that longer and/or faster NSVT may also affect the risk of SD (Gersh et al. 2011).

Viswanathan (Viswanathan et al. 2016) analyzed the relationship between rapid NSVT (RNSVT) detected by ICD within 12 months of implant, defined as 4-16 beats at ≥150-200 bpm and a major risk factor for sudden cardiac death in hypertrophic cardiomyopathy. The authors suggested that Rapid NSVT detected by continuous monitoring independently predicted ventricular arrhythmia in HCM and offered superior discrimination of ventricular arrhythmia risk compared to conventional risk factors, including Holter-NSVT.

Francia (Francia et al. 2014) confirmed that ICD-NSVT compared to Holter recordings in the same patients was longer and significantly faster, often exceeding 200 bpm. Of note, ICD-NSVT was faster than Holter-NSVT in virtually all patients. Taken together, these results suggest that in HCM patients long-lasting and rapid NSVTs are less common than slow and relatively short NSVTs. Nonetheless, rapid-rate and prolonged NSVT predict the risk of life-threatening arrhythmias. Accordingly, the finding of slow and short-lasting NSVT on Holter ECG in a given patient with established major risk factors for SD may be only partially representative of the global arrhythmic burden. Francia (Francia et al. 2014) proposed that a simple index of NSVT severity (heart rate × length in beats/100>28) predicted ICD intervention.

Future studies are needed to validate these findings in a larger HCM cohort.

Family History of Sudden Cardiac Death at a Young Age

While it has been recognized that SCD events can cluster in families, the data is somewhat conflicting regarding the link between family history of SCD and risk for any individual patient. This is likely related to differences in the definition of familial SCD in the various studies.

Notably, most studies have used 40–50 as an age cut-off and have considered only first-degree relatives (P. Elliott et al. 2006; Christiaans et al. 2010; Maki et al. 1998; P. Spirito et al. 2000; P. M. Elliott et al. 2000; Bos et al. 2010).

Several studies have been unable to demonstrate a significant relationship between family history of SCD and SCD on multivariable analysis (P. M. Elliott et al. 2000; Bos et al. 2010). A recent meta-analysis, on the other hand, has demonstrated an independent but weak correlation, with an average reported hazard ratio of 1.27 (Christiaans et al. 2010).

Syncope

Syncope occurs in 15–25% of patients with HCM (P. M. Elliott et al. 2000) with the principal causes being broadly divided into two mechanistic categories: (i) arrhythmic causes (both brady- and tachyarrhythmias) and (ii) primary hemodynamic abnormalities such as left ventricular outflow tract obstruction (LVOTO) and abnormal vascular control mechanisms.

Given the multifactorial etiologies for syncope, a thorough clinical history is required before it can be considered a potential marker for sudden death.

The most compelling data relating unexplained syncope with increased risk of sudden death comes from a large consecutive series of 1511 patients. In this cohort, the relative risk of SCD was 1.78 in those patients with a history of recurrent syncope compared with patients without such a history (Paolo Spirito et al. 2009).

This association held true only when syncope had occurred within the preceding 6 months. In patients with a remote history of syncope (>5 years prior to the clinical visit), no independent association with SCD could be demonstrated.

Exercise Blood Pressure Response

An abnormal blood pressure response is present in up to one-third of patients with HCM (Frenneaux et al. 1990; I. Olivotto et al. 1999). Possible mechanisms for abnormal blood pressure response include LV outflow tract obstruction leading to a fall in cardiac output, inadequate diastolic filling time at high heart rates leading to a fall in stroke volume, and a fall in systemic vascular resistance due to inappropriate vasodilatation (Frenneaux et al. 1990; Ciampi et al. 2002; Counihan et al. 1991).

Furthermore, HCM patients with abnormal blood pressure response have only a marginally lower exercise duration than do subjects with a normal blood pressure response. Yet, in contrast, these patients demonstrate a dramatically lower cardiac output response (Campbell et al. 2003).

Abnormal blood pressure response is noted more often in younger patients, and in those with a family history of HCM or sudden death (Frenneaux et al. 1990). The presence of abnormal blood pressure response has been associated with an increased risk of sudden death in patients below the age of 50 (with an odds ratio of 4.5 in one study) (I. Olivotto et al. 1999), albeit with a very low positive predictive value of 14–15% (I. Olivotto et al. 1999; Sadoul et al. 1997). However, the high negative predictive value of 95–97% means that its absence is potentially useful in reassuring the patient in the absence of any other risk factors for SCD (I. Olivotto et al. 1999; Sadoul et al. 1997).

Interestingly, a recent study of 426 asymptomatic or minimally symptomatic patients with HCM highlighted that exercise capacity and not blood pressure response was an independent predictor for adverse outcomes. Patients achieving 100% of predicted METs had a low rate event of 1% compared with 12% in those achieving 85% of predicted METs (Desai et al. 2014).

Potential Risk Modifiers

Risk modifiers can be used in conjunction with established risk markers to determine a patient's risk of SCD (Gersh et al. 2011). Risk modifiers include late gadolinium enhancement (LGE) on cardiac magnetic resonance imaging (cMRI), LV apical aneurysm and genetic mutations.

Late Gadolinium Enhancement on Cardiac Magnetic Resonance Imaging

Since the 1970s, echocardiography has been established as the gold standard diagnostic tool in HCM (Barry J. Maron et al. 2014). With the development of cMRI in the 1980s, this imaging modality has assumed an important role in characterizing variations in HCM morphology and function, distinguishing it from other cardiomyopathies, stratifying risk, and guiding treatment.

Disertori (Disertori, Masè, and Ravelli 2017) demonstrated that myocardial fibrosis is a common pattern in the setting of different heart diseases, and promotes ventricular tachyarrhythmias by creating a vulnerable substrate for reentrant activity and by favoring the emergence of triggers.

The use of contrast cardiac magnetic resonance (CMR) imaging with late gadolinium enhancement (LGE) has enabled us to identify and quantify myocardial fibrosis in a non-invasive way. The histological basis of LGE in HCM has traditionally been difficult to assess, but a strong correlation was previously demonstrated between the extent of myocardial fibrosis in LV myocardium obtained from septal myectomy (as assessed by histologic examination) and LGE (as determined from contrast-enhanced CMR studies performed prior to myectomy) (Moravsky et al. 2013). Currently, cMRI is being used to better understand the role of fibrosis and how it relates to disease progression and risk of SCD (Briasoulis et al. 2015). Extensive fibrosis is a common finding at postmortem examination of patients who have died suddenly (Basso et al. 2000). Fibrosis is also associated with systolic dysfunction and heart failure (M. S. Maron, Appelbaum, et al. 2008).

Of note, regions of late enhancement can represent partial rather than complete replacement fibrosis (Moon et al. 2004). The amount of LGE can be quantified as a percentage of the total LV mass. About two-thirds of patients with HCM display areas of LGE in varying degrees of extent and location. In HCM patients, dense areas of replacement fibrosis are usually present in hypertrophied regions involving the mid-myocardial wall, with a patchy multifocal distribution, or located at the junctional areas between the right and the left ventricle (van der Bijl, Delgado, et Bax 2016).

Data on LGE prognostic values for ventricular arrhythmias is less uniform in HCM patients than in other cardiomyopathies. The first meta-analysis on 1,063 HCM patients by Green in 2012 (Green et al. 2012) suggested a trend for LGE predictive power for SCD events, without reaching statistical significance. Several studies have demonstrated a strong association between the presence of LGE and increased ventricular ectopy and NSVT on ambulatory Holter monitoring (Adabag et al. 2008; Kwon et al. 2008; Rubinshtein et al. 2010; Inada et al. 2011).

As NSVT is an independent predictor of SCD, this has led to the investigation of the relationship between LGE and SCD, and its potential role as a novel risk factor.

While most studies have found LGE to be a univariate predictor of SCD, findings regarding LGE as an independent predictor for SCD are inconsistent. The predictive power of LGE extent for SCD events was recently analyzed in detail by Chan et al. (Chan et al. 2014). In this large, multi-center study of 1,293 HCM patients with low arrhythmic risk according to conventional risk factors (60% with zero risk factor, and 32% with one risk factor), LGE emerged as an independent predictor for SCD, where there was a continuous relationship between the extent of LGE and the risk of SCD. Tachyarrhythmic events occurred in 3% of the patients during a median follow-up of 3.3 years. The incidence of SCD per 1,000 person-year was directly proportional to the percentage extent of LGE, increasing from 4 per 1,000 person-year in the absence of LGE, to 10 at LGE ≤10%, 18 at 11-19% LGE, and 24 at LGE ≥20% (Chan et al. 2014).

Similarly, a recent meta-analysis by Weng (Weng et al. 2016) which included an enlarged population of 2,993 HCM patients, robustly showed LGE predictive power for SCD with an odds ratio of 3.41. Both the presence and extent of LGE appeared to be strong independent predictors of SCD in HCM patients, even after adjusting for baseline characteristics. The quantification of LGE extent instead of LGE presence may be more useful clinically because up to 70% of HCM patients display some degree of LGE on CMR. Amano (Amano et al. 2017) showed on 115 patients with HCM and LGE that the clinical and MRI findings of the patients with HCM and ventricular tachyarrhythmia were distinct from those of patients without ventricular tachyarrhythmia. The amount of nonseptal LGE was significantly related to the serious arrhythmia associated with HCM and to ICD implantation. By contrast, septal LGE was not related to ventricular tachyarrhythmia in patients with HCM and LGE. Thus, paying more attention to the extent of nonseptal LGE is essential for risk stratification of HCM associated with myocardial scarring. In addition, the number of nonseptal LGE segments was significantly greater in the HCM patients with myocardial scarring (i.e., LGE) and ventricular tachyarrhythmia (mean, 3.3 segments) than in those with scarring but no tachyarrhythmia (mean, 1.7 segments). There was a significant correlation between the extent of nonseptal LGE and that of global LGE, and multivariate analysis revealed that the extent of nonseptal LGE was related to the episode of ventricular tachyarrhythmia in addition to the number of clinical risk markers. In the present study, myocardial LGE extent was assessed based on the AHA 17-segment model but not the mass of LGE, partly because the mass may not necessarily reflect the location and dispersion of the scarring. A substantial extent of myocardial fibrosis (≥15% of total LV mass) was associated with a two-fold increase in SCD at 5 years compared with patients with no LGE (Chan et al. 2014). In contrast, a study by Ismail et al. on 711 patients who were followed for a median of 3.5 years found the amount of LGE to be significantly associated with SCD on univariable regression. However, the association did not remain statistically significant after adjustment for LV ejection fraction (Ismail et al. 2014).

A recent meta-analysis of six clinical studies has shown that LGE is significantly correlated with increased risk of SCD in low-risk patients according to conventional risk factors (Briasoulis et al. 2015). Notably, only the presence, but not the extent of LGE, was significantly related to the risk of SCD. A recent study showed that hinge point LGE is not a determinant of SCD risk (Chan et al. 2015). Interestingly, the spatial distribution of LGE significantly correlated with depolarizing and repolarizing electrical abnormalities in high-risk patients with malignant ventricular arrhythmia (N. Sakamoto et al. 2015). Recently, Hinojar (Hinojar et al. 2017) showed that LGE extension is concordant with the SCD-risk model proposed by current ESC guidelines. Although only a minority of patients at low risk exhibited extensive areas of LGE, nearly all of the patients in the high-risk group showed ≥15% LGE. All patients in the intermediate- and high-risk groups showed any amount of LGE, suggesting that its absence could identify low-risk patients, but its presence per se is not enough to define risk. Their findings suggest an additive role of LGE imaging as an arbitrator after clinical risk assessment, particularly when an intermediate risk is estimated (Hinojar et al. 2017). Doesch (Doesch et al. 2017) showed that HCM patients with a high risk of SCD according to the ESC clinical risk prediction model revealed the highest extent of LGE % compared to patients with HCM and lower ESC risk scores. The extent LGE % showed a better predictive value to estimate major adverse cardiac arrhythmic events than ESC risk score. Furthermore, in patients with a low and intermediate ESC risk score <6%, a high extent LGE % identified a subgroup of patients with an increased risk for major adverse cardiac arrhythmic events. On the other hand, in patients with a high ESC risk score ≥6%, an extent LGE <20% was associated with a low risk of major adverse cardiac arrhythmic events. Therefore, these results support the hypothesis that the extent of LGE may play a role as an additional risk marker that could help further improve risk stratification in these patients.

SCD in HCM is assumed to originate from the myocardial disarray and scar tissue (P. M. Elliott et al. 2000; Stroumpoulis, Pantazopoulos, et Xanthos 2010), which is, for example, more present in patients with increased LVWT. Several studies have shown that the presence of extensive fibrosis, demonstrated by LGE on cMRI, might increase the risk of SCD (Olivotto et al. 2010; Chan et al. 2014; Ismail et al. 2014; Adabag et al. 2008), but a recent meta-analysis did not show any relationship with SCD (Green et al. 2012). There is a relationship however between extensive delayed enhancement and progression to heart failure (Bruder et al. 2010).

Extensive LGE, comprising ≥15% of total LV mass, prospectively identifies patients with preserved systolic function who are at risk of heart failure progression due to systolic dysfunction and who may require future heart transplantation (Chan et al. 2014). The prognosis of Dilated HCM is very poor, and heart failure and sudden cardiac death are the main causes of death.

LV Apical Aneurysms (Detailed in Chapter 6)

Genetics of Hypertrophic Cardiomyopathy

Currently, there is minimal evidence to support the use of genetic testing to identify patients who are at high risk of SCD. Small studies have found that patients with a more malignant inheritance of their mutations (i.e., homozygous mutations) as well as the presence of a *MYH7* gene mutation have increased rates of heart failure (Barry J. Maron, Maron, et Semsarian 2012). Emerging data suggests that rarer forms of the *MYH7* mutation increase the risk of SCD (Barry J. Maron, Maron, et Semsarian 2012; Wang et al. 2014). However, Chida (Chida et al. 2017) showed that those with *MYH7* and *MYBPC3* mutations did not have a significantly different prognosis compared with non-mutation carriers, but the rate of ventricular arrhythmia and/or past history of syncope was the highest in

MYBPC3 mutation carriers among these three groups; as such, *MYBPC3* patients should be followed closely based on the possibility of SD.

Ingles (Ingles et al. 2005) describe the frequency of single and multiple gene mutations in an Australian cohort of 80 unrelated HCM families. A gene mutation was identified in 23 probands (29%), with four probands being compound or double heterozygote genotypes (5%). Probands carrying multiple gene mutations were shown to express a more severe clinical phenotype than single heterozygote HCM patients, as demonstrated by an increase in left ventricular hypertrophy and an increased incidence of sudden cardiac death events.

Despite rapid development and utilization of genetic testing, specific recommendations for clinical implication were not addressed in 2011 but are an important consideration and option in managing HCM patients (Fraiche and Wang 2016). In the recent 2014 European Society of Cardiology (ESC) HCM Guidelines, algorithms were proposed for 3 categories of genetic test results—definite mutations, variants of unknown significance, and no mutation—to evaluate patients diagnosed with HCM and first-degree relatives. However, current recommendations for genetic testing remain limited to screening rather than advocating it for risk stratification (Authors/Task Force members et al. 2014).

Models for Estimating Sudden Cardiac Death Risk

Sudden cardiac death (SCD) may complicate the natural course of hypertrophic cardiomyopathy (HCM). Selecting patients for implantable cardioverter defibrillator (ICD) therapy in the primary prevention setting is still a challenge.

Originally in the 2003 ACC/ESC guidelines and 2011 ACCF/AHA guidelines, the identification of high-risk patients was based on five clinical characteristics: a family history of SCD in first-degree relatives < 40 years of age, maximal left ventricular wall thickness (LVWT) >30 mm, unexplainable syncope, non-sustained ventricular tachycardia (NSVT) and abnormal blood pressure response during exercise (Barry J. Maron et al. 2003; Gersh et al. 2011). In the 2011 ACCF/AHA guidelines, the clinical variables are grouped into two categories where the first category includes established risk markers. Some of these markers are individually sufficient to prompt ICD placement, while others prompt ICD placement when found in conjunction with other high-risk factors. The second category includes risk modifiers. These serve as additional markers to help identify high-risk patients; alone they are not sufficient to promote ICD placement. Established risk markers carry more weight, as the evidence linking them to SCD is more robust (Gersh et al. 2011).

Although it was clear that the risk of SCD increases with increasing number of risk factors, O'Mahony (O'Mahony et al. 2013) demonstrated that both the 2003 and 2011 guidelines distinguish high and low risk patients with only limited power. Recently the HCM Outcome Investigators presented a novel clinical risk prediction model for SCD (HCM Risk-SCD), based on a cohort of 3,675 patients from six centers (O'Mahony et al. 2014). This model provides an individualized 5-year risk, based on most of the aforementioned risk factors, combined with left ventricular outflow tract (LVOT) gradient, left atrial (LA) diameter, and age at evaluation. This new model was more accurate in predicting SCD compared with the conventional risk factors, and the recently released 2014 ESC guidelines incorporated the HCM Risk-SCD model to classify patients as low risk (5-year risk of SCD <4%), intermediate risk (5-year risk of SCD 4-6%) or high risk (5-year risk of SCD >6%). ICD implantation was a IIb or IIa recommendation in the latter groups, respectively.

This model calculates individual 5-year SCD risk estimates. Their results show that, in an independent setting, the ability to predict SCD by using the HCM Risk-SCD model (C-statistic = 0.69) is improved when compared with current guidelines (C-statistic = 0.55-0.60).

This HCM Risk-SCD is calculated as follows: Probability SCD at 5 years = 1 – 0.998 exp (Prognostic index), where Prognostic index = (0.15939858 x maximal wall thickness (mm)) - (0.00294271 x maximal wall thickness^2 (mm^2)) + (0.0259082 x left atrial diameter (mm)) +

(0.00446131 x maximal (rest/Valsalva) left ventricular outflow tract gradient (mm Hg)) + (0.4583082 x family history SCD) + (0.82639195 x NSVT) + (0.71650361 x unexplained syncope) - (0.01799934 x age at clinical evaluation (years)).

There are no randomized trials or statistically validated prospective prediction models that can be used to guide ICD implantation in patients with HCM. Recommendations are instead based on observational, retrospective cohort studies that have determined the relationship between clinical characteristics and prognosis (Authors/Task Force members et al. 2014).

In O'Mahony's study (O'Mahony et al. 2014), HCM Risk-SCD uses predictor variables that have been associated with an increased risk of sudden death in at least one published multivariable analysis. The model provides individualized 5-year risk estimates and, in a head to head comparison with a model using four major risk factors, the performance of the prediction model improved substantially (C-index from 0.54 to 0.7).

The biggest changes in the HCM Risk-SCD model, compared with the risk stratification models proposed by the older guidelines, are the following: (1) abnormal blood pressure response during exercise is no longer included in the risk stratification; (2) increasing age is a protective factor; (3) LVWT is no longer regarded as dichotomous, but as a continuous variable; and (4) LA diameter and LVOT gradient are added as continuous risk factors. All clinical variables are easily obtained, especially since abnormal blood pressure response during exercise is no longer a risk factor. Although there was a univariable association between blood pressure response and SCD (Sadoul et al. 1997), it remained unclear if it was only of clinical importance in patients $\leq$40 years old (P. M. Elliott et al. 2000), or how the finding was related to the increase in dynamic LVOT gradient.

In the 2011 guidelines, the usefulness of ICD implantation in the presence of an abnormal blood pressure response as the only risk factor was deemed uncertain (Class IIb, level of evidence C)(Gersh et al. 2011), and it was excluded as a potential risk factor in the HCM Risk-SCD model because it was not associated with SCD in any multivariable survival analyses (P. M. Elliott et al. 2000; Gimeno et al. 2009; Efthimiadis et al. 2009).

Age is considered to be protective of SCD in this model. A number of studies have demonstrated that a younger age is associated with an increased risk of SCD (Maki et al. 1998; Paolo Spirito et al. 2009), and a recent study showed a very low SCD risk in patients >60 years of age (Barry J. Maron et al. 2013).

Another advantage of the new model is that the effects of cardiac remodeling on SCD are now taken into consideration. HCM is not a static disease and Olivotto et al. identified 4 clinical stages of HCM and demonstrated that disease progression is associated with an increase of SCD risk: from 0.5%-1%/year in patients with classic phenotype to 10%/year in patients with overt dysfunction (Olivotto et al. 2012). This increase of risk is not taken into consideration in conventional risk prediction models.

The new HCM Risk-SCD model is partially based on factors of disease progression including maximal LVWT, LA diameter and LVOT gradient. These factors are, as mentioned above, included in the model as continuous variables, and changes therein are reflected in the SCD risk score.

In order to validate this risk calculator, the estimated risk of SCD was examined retrospectively in a cohort of 1,629 patients with HCM. The investigators compared the calculated risk of SCD with the actual event rate over long-term follow-up (Barry J. Maron, Casey, et al. 2015). The results showed a significant underestimation of SCD risk by the ESC risk model, with only 11% of the 35 patients who had a SCD event considered at high risk and for whom ICD would be recommended; and 60% of the patients who experienced a clinical SCD event were calculated to have a low risk (<4% annual risk) and with ICD not recommended (Fraiche and Wang 2016). Zhonghua (Zhu et al. 2017) showed in Chinese patients that the predicted rate of an SCD event calculated by HCM Risk-SCD was lower than the actual rate of SCD, but that prediction efficiency and indication for ICD implantation of HCM Risk-SCD were better than those from the 2011 AHA guideline. Fernandez (Fernández et al. 2016) showed that the new model proved to be an excellent predictor because the area under the curve for estimated risk was 0.925 in patients from South America. Vriesendorp (Vriesendorp et al. 2015) showed the HCM Risk-SCD score discriminated better between patients with high or low SCD risk than the risk stratification models proposed by older clinical guidelines.

The HCM Risk-SCD model improves the risk stratification of HCM patients, and calculating an individual risk estimate contributes to the clinical decision-making process. Improved risk stratification is important for making a decision before ICD implantation for primary prevention of SCD.

In addition, it is unclear how septal reduction therapy (both surgical myectomy and septal ablation) influences individual SCD risk, and whether or not it is sufficient to calculate the new 5-year risk by using the post-procedural LVOT gradient and LVWT. Several studies demonstrated that SCD rates after myectomy are low, but the SCD risk after septal ablation is more controversial (Ommen et al. 2005; ten Cate et al. 2010; Veselka, Tomašov, et Zemánek 2011; Jensen et al. 2013).

Cardiopulmonary exercise testing can also be useful in stratifying risk in hypertrophic cardiomyopathy (Finocchiaro et al. 2015; Belardinelli et al. 2003; Masri et al. 2015; Coats et al. 2015; Magrì et al. 2016). A recent study by Magri (Magrì et al. 2016) on 623 patients (3.7 yr median follow-up, 25 events) identified a VE/VCO2 slope value greater than 31 as the only cardiopulmonary exercise test variable to be independently associated with sudden cardiac death. This parameter might improve SCD risk stratification, particularly in those HCM categories classified as low-intermediate SCD risk according to contemporary guidelines.

Some electrocardiographic parameters may be useful for risk stratification in patients with HCM. They were recently described in Akboğa's study (Akboğa et al. 2017) which showed that the Tp-e interval and Tp-e/QTc ratio were significantly longer and higher in patients with HCM and were associated with a higher risk of ventricular arrhythmic events.

Several biomarkers have been also studied in HCM, including natriuretic peptides, neutrophil-to-lymphocyte ratio and matrix metalloproteinases (Brito 2017; Cambronero et al. 2009; EXpert Group on Biomarkers 2014; Münch et al. 2016).

It is important to note that our current understanding is still incomplete. As always, a decision must be tailored to the needs and desires of the individual patient.

Implantable Cardioverter Defibrillators and HCM

The use of implantable cardioverter defibrillators (ICDs) for primary prevention of SCD in patients with clinical risk factors has improved the survival of patients with HCM (Barry J. Maron, Rowin, et al. 2015). High risk patients can be protected from SCD by implantable cardioverter-defibrillators (ICD), but this protection comes at the price of inappropriate shocks and device-related complications (Schinkel et al. 2012).

Maron (Barry J. Maron et al. 2007) developed complications of ICD in the study of 506 patients, where 136 (27%) experienced one or more inappropriate shocks due to sinus tachycardia, atrial fibrillation, or lead malfunction. Major complications included infection in 19 (3.8%), hemorrhage/thrombosis in 8 (1.6%), and lead fractures, dislodgement, and oversensing in 34 (6.7%). Inappropriate shocks occurred with similar frequency in both primary (25%) and secondary prevention patients (32%) (P=.38) and were no more common in patients 30 years old or younger (32%) than in those older than 30 (23%) (P=.22).

Beta-blocker therapy was associated with fewer inappropriate ICD interventions (Konstantinou et al. 2016).

In order to limit ICD complication like inappropriate shocks, the four continental electrophysiology societies (Wilkoff et al. 2016) proposed focused recommendations for ICD programming with a long overdue effort to provide analysis and guidance to the clinician as to how to make strategic programming choices in implementing ICD therapy. There are hundreds of choices for which there is inadequate data to provide evidence or consensus-based recommendations. The discussion and recommendations have been limited here to four areas for which there was sufficient consensus and data. Many questions have been intentionally left unanswered.

However, the best tool to limit ICD complications is to improve clinical risk stratification.

CONCLUSION

Sudden cardiac death events in HCM patients occur unpredictably, often without warning signs or symptoms and are most common in young people through mid-life. Using ICD for primary prevention of sudden death in HCM has created the opportunity to prevent these catastrophic events, but this protection comes at the price of complications. This has placed increased importance on risk stratification to help identify individuals who may benefit from device therapy for primary prevention.

Several parameters have been developed and established as risk factors and some are integrated into a risk-prediction scoring system. However, these parameters have limitations in sensitivity and specificity.

These models must be further studied and refined for worldwide HCM populations. Future algorithms should include older risk modifiers and eventually new parameters on electrocardiogram, cardiopulmonary exercise testing and biomarkers.

REFERENCES

Adabag, A. Selcuk, Susan A. Casey, Michael A. Kuskowski, Andrey G. Zenovich, et Barry J. Maron. 2005. "Spectrum and Prognostic Significance of Arrhythmias on Ambulatory Holter Electrocardiogram in Hypertrophic Cardiomyopathy." *Journal of the American College of Cardiology* 45 (5): 697‑704. doi:10.1016/j.jacc.2004.11.043.

Adabag, A. Selcuk, Barry J. Maron, Evan Appelbaum, Caitlin J. Harrigan, Jacqueline L. Buros, C. Michael Gibson, John R. Lesser, et al. 2008.

"Occurrence and Frequency of Arrhythmias in Hypertrophic Cardiomyopathy in Relation to Delayed Enhancement on Cardiovascular Magnetic Resonance." *Journal of the American College of Cardiology* 51 (14): 1369‑74. doi:10.1016/j.jacc.2007.11.071.

Akboğa, Mehmet Kadri, Kevser Gülcihan Balcı, Samet Yılmaz, Selahattin Aydın, Çağrı Yayla, Ahmet Göktuğ Ertem, Sefa Ünal, et al. 2017. "Tp-e Interval and Tp-e/QTc Ratio as Novel Surrogate Markers for Prediction of Ventricular Arrhythmic Events in Hypertrophic Cardiomyopathy." *Anatolian Journal of Cardiology* 18 (1): 48‑53. doi:10.14744/AnatolJCardiol.2017.7581.

Amano, Yasuo, Fumi Yanagisawa, Mitsunobu Kitamura, Masaki Tachi, et Shinichiro Kumita. 2017. "Relationship of Nonseptal Late Gadolinium Enhancement to Ventricular Tachyarrhythmia in Hypertrophic Cardiomyopathy." *Journal of Computer Assisted Tomography*, juillet. doi:10.1097/RCT.0000000000000599.

Authors/Task Force members, Perry M. Elliott, Aris Anastasakis, Michael A. Borger, Martin Borggrefe, Franco Cecchi, Philippe Charron, et al. 2014. "2014 ESC Guidelines on Diagnosis and Management of Hypertrophic Cardiomyopathy: The Task Force for the Diagnosis and Management of Hypertrophic Cardiomyopathy of the European Society of Cardiology (ESC)." *European Heart Journal* 35 (39): 2733‑79. doi:10.1093/eurheartj/ehu284.

Basso, C., G. Thiene, D. Corrado, G. Buja, P. Melacini, et A. Nava. 2000. "Hypertrophic Cardiomyopathy and Sudden Death in the Young: Pathologic Evidence of Myocardial Ischemia." *Human Pathology* 31 (8): 988‑98. doi:10.1053/hupa.2000.16659.

Belardinelli, Romualdo, Francesca Lacalaprice, Flavia Carle, Adelaide Minnucci, Giovanni Cianci, GianPiero Perna, et Giuseppe D'Eusanio. 2003. "Exercise-Induced Myocardial Ischaemia Detected by Cardiopulmonary Exercise Testing." *European Heart Journal* 24 (14): 1304‑13.

Betensky, Brian P., et Sanjay Dixit. 2014. "Sudden Cardiac Death in Patients with Nonischemic Cardiomyopathy." *Indian Heart Journal* 66 (janvier): S35‑45. doi:10.1016/j.ihj.2013.12.047.

Bijl, Pieter van der, Victoria Delgado, et Jeroen J. Bax. 2016. "Noninvasive Imaging Markers Associated with Sudden Cardiac Death." *Trends in Cardiovascular Medicine* 26 (4): 348‑60. doi:10.1016/j.tcm.2015.10.003.

Borggrefe, M., H. Kuhn, H. H. Königer, H. Stöter, G. Breithardt, F. Loogen, H. D. Schulte, et W. Bircks. 1983. "Arrhythmias in Hypertrophic Obstructive and Non-Obstructive Cardiomyopathy." *European Heart Journal* 4 Suppl F (novembre): 245‑51.

Bos, J. Martijn, Barry J. Maron, Michael J. Ackerman, Tammy S. Haas, Paul Sorajja, Rick A. Nishimura, Bernard J. Gersh, et Steve R. Ommen. 2010. "Role of Family History of Sudden Death in Risk Stratification and Prevention of Sudden Death with Implantable Defibrillators in Hypertrophic Cardiomyopathy." *The American Journal of Cardiology* 106 (10): 1481‑86. doi:10.1016/j.amjcard.2010.06.077.

Briasoulis, Alexandros, Sagar Mallikethi-Reddy, Mohan Palla, Issa Alesh, et Luis Afonso. 2015. "Myocardial Fibrosis on Cardiac Magnetic Resonance and Cardiac Outcomes in Hypertrophic Cardiomyopathy: A Meta-Analysis." *Heart (British Cardiac Society)* 101 (17): 1406‑11. doi:10.1136/heartjnl-2015-307682.

Brito, Dulce. 2017. "Predicting Risk of Sudden Death in Hypertrophic Cardiomyopathy: Can Additional Simple Markers Help?" *Revista Portuguesa De Cardiologia: Orgao Oficial Da Sociedade Portuguesa De Cardiologia = Portuguese Journal of Cardiology: An Official Journal of the Portuguese Society of Cardiology* 36 (4): 247‑49. doi:10.1016/j.repc.2017.02.005.

Brito, Dulce, J. Sampaio Matias, Luís Sargento, Maria João Cabral, et Hugo C. Madeira. 2004. "Plasma N-Terminal pro-Brain Natriuretic Peptide: A Marker of Left Ventricular Hypertrophy in Hypertrophic Cardiomyopathy." *Revista Portuguesa De Cardiologia: Orgao Oficial Da Sociedade Portuguesa De Cardiologia = Portuguese Journal of*

Cardiology: An Official Journal of the Portuguese Society of Cardiology 23 (12): 1557‑82.

Bruder, Oliver, Anja Wagner, Christoph J. Jensen, Steffen Schneider, Peter Ong, Eva-Maria Kispert, Kai Nassenstein, et al. 2010. "Myocardial Scar Visualized by Cardiovascular Magnetic Resonance Imaging Predicts Major Adverse Events in Patients with Hypertrophic Cardiomyopathy." *Journal of the American College of Cardiology* 56 (11): 875‑87. doi:10.1016/j.jacc.2010.05.007.

Cambronero, Francisco, Francisco Marín, Vanessa Roldán, Diana Hernández-Romero, Mariano Valdés, et Gregory Y. H. Lip. 2009. "Biomarkers of Pathophysiology in Hypertrophic Cardiomyopathy: Implications for Clinical Management and Prognosis." *European Heart Journal* 30 (2): 139‑51. doi:10.1093/eurheartj/ehn538.

Campbell, Ross, Dante E Manyari, William J McKenna, et Michael Frenneaux. 2003. "What is the mechanism of abnormal blood pressure response on exercise in hypertrophic cardiomyopathy?" *Journal of the American College of Cardiology* 41 (11): 2102. doi:10.1016/S0735-1097(03)00364-4.

Castro-Torres, Yaniel. 2017. "Tp-e Interval and Tp-e/QTc Ratio: New Choices for Risk Stratification of Arrhythmic Events in Patients with Hypertrophic Cardiomyopathy." *Anatolian Journal of Cardiology* 17 (6): 493.

Cate, Folkert J. ten, Osama I. I. Soliman, Michelle Michels, Dominic A. M. J. Theuns, Peter L. de Jong, Marcel L. Geleijnse, et Patrick W. Serruys. 2010. "Long-Term Outcome of Alcohol Septal Ablation in Patients with Obstructive Hypertrophic Cardiomyopathy: A Word of Caution." *Circulation. Heart Failure* 3 (3): 362‑69. doi:10.1161/CIRCHEARTFAILURE.109.862359.

Chan, Raymond H., Barry J. Maron, Iacopo Olivotto, Gabriele E. Assenza, Tammy S. Haas, John R. Lesser, Christiane Gruner, et al. 2015. "Significance of Late Gadolinium Enhancement at Right Ventricular Attachment to Ventricular Septum in Patients with Hypertrophic Cardiomyopathy." *The American Journal of Cardiology* 116 (3): 436‑41. doi:10.1016/j.amjcard.2015.04.060.

Chan, Raymond H., Barry J. Maron, Iacopo Olivotto, Michael J. Pencina, Gabriele Egidy Assenza, Tammy Haas, John R. Lesser, et al. 2014. "Prognostic Value of Quantitative Contrast-Enhanced Cardiovascular Magnetic Resonance for the Evaluation of Sudden Death Risk in Patients with Hypertrophic Cardiomyopathy." *Circulation* 130 (6): 484‑95. doi:10.1161/CIRCULATIONAHA.113.007094.

Chida, Ayako, Kei Inai, Hiroki Sato, Eriko Shimada, Tsutomu Nishizawa, Mitsuyo Shimada, Michiko Furutani, et al. 2017. "Prognostic Predictive Value of Gene Mutations in Japanese Patients with Hypertrophic Cardiomyopathy." *Heart and Vessels* 32 (6): 700‑707. doi:10.1007/s00380-016-0920-0.

Christiaans, Imke, Klaartje van Engelen, Irene M. van Langen, Erwin Birnie, Gouke J. Bonsel, Perry M. Elliott, et Arthur A. M. Wilde. 2010. "Risk Stratification for Sudden Cardiac Death in Hypertrophic Cardiomyopathy: Systematic Review of Clinical Risk Markers." *Europace: European Pacing, Arrhythmias, and Cardiac Electrophysiology: Journal of the Working Groups on Cardiac Pacing, Arrhythmias, and Cardiac Cellular Electrophysiology of the European Society of Cardiology* 12 (3): 313‑21. doi:10.1093/europace/eup431.

Ciampi, Quirino, Sandro Betocchi, Raffaella Lombardi, Fiore Manganelli, Giovanni Storto, Maria Angela Losi, Elpidio Pezzella, Filippo Finizio, Alberto Cuocolo, et Massimo Chiariello. 2002. "Hemodynamic Determinants of Exercise-Induced Abnormal Blood Pressure Response in Hypertrophic Cardiomyopathy." *Journal of the American College of Cardiology* 40 (2): 278‑84.

Coats, Caroline J., Khadija Rantell, Aleksandra Bartnik, Amour Patel, Bryan Mist, William J. McKenna, et Perry M. Elliott. 2015. "Cardiopulmonary Exercise Testing and Prognosis in Hypertrophic Cardiomyopathy." *Circulation. Heart Failure* 8 (6): 1022‑31. doi:10.1161/CIRCHEARTFAILURE.114.002248.

Counihan, P. J., M. P. Frenneaux, D. J. Webb, et W. J. McKenna. 1991. "Abnormal Vascular Responses to Supine Exercise in Hypertrophic Cardiomyopathy." *Circulation* 84 (2): 686‑96.

Desai, Milind Y., Aditya Bhonsale, Parag Patel, Peyman Naji, Nicholas G. Smedira, Maran Thamilarasan, Bruce W. Lytle, et Harry M. Lever. 2014. "Exercise Echocardiography in Asymptomatic HCM: Exercise Capacity, and Not LV Outflow Tract Gradient Predicts Long-Term Outcomes." *JACC. Cardiovascular Imaging* 7 (1): 26-36. doi:10.1016/j.jcmg.2013.08.010.

Dimitrow, Pawel Petkow, Lidia Chojnowska, Tomasz Rudzinski, Walerian Piotrowski, Lidia Ziólkowska, Andrzej Wojtarowicz, Anna Wycisk, et al. 2010. "Sudden Death in Hypertrophic Cardiomyopathy: Old Risk Factors Re-Assessed in a New Model of Maximalized Follow-Up." *European Heart Journal* 31 (24): 3084-93. doi:10.1093/eurheartj/ehq308.

Disertori, Marcello, Michela Masè, et Flavia Ravelli. 2017. "Myocardial Fibrosis Predicts Ventricular Tachyarrhythmias." *Trends in Cardiovascular Medicine* 27 (5): 363-72. doi:10.1016/j.tcm.2017.01.011.

Doesch, Christina, Erol Tülümen, Ibrahim Akin, Boris Rudic, Juergen Kuschyk, Ibrahim El-Battrawy, Tobias Becher, et al. 2017. "Incremental Benefit of Late Gadolinium Cardiac Magnetic Resonance Imaging for Risk Stratification in Patients with Hypertrophic Cardiomyopathy." *Scientific Reports* 7 (1): 6336. doi:10.1038/s41598-017-06533-0.

Efthimiadis, Georgios K., Despina G. Parcharidou, Georgios Giannakoulas, Efstathios D. Pagourelias, Panagiotis Charalampidis, Gregorios Savvopoulos, Antonios Ziakas, Haralambos Karvounis, Ioannis H. Styliadis, et Georgios E. Parcharidis. 2009. "Left Ventricular Outflow Tract Obstruction as a Risk Factor for Sudden Cardiac Death in Hypertrophic Cardiomyopathy." *The American Journal of Cardiology* 104 (5): 695-99. doi:10.1016/j.amjcard.2009.04.039.

Elliott, P. M., J. R. Gimeno Blanes, N. G. Mahon, J. D. Poloniecki, et W. J. McKenna. 2001. "Relation between Severity of Left-Ventricular Hypertrophy and Prognosis in Patients with Hypertrophic

Cardiomyopathy." *Lancet (London, England)* 357 (9254): 420‑24. doi:10.1016/S0140-6736(00)04005-8.

Elliott, P. M., J. Poloniecki, S. Dickie, S. Sharma, L. Monserrat, A. Varnava, N. G. Mahon, et W. J. McKenna. 2000. "Sudden Death in Hypertrophic Cardiomyopathy: Identification of High Risk Patients." *Journal of the American College of Cardiology* 36 (7): 2212‑18.

Elliott, P. M., S. Sharma, A. Varnava, J. Poloniecki, E. Rowland, et W. J. McKenna. 1999. "Survival after Cardiac Arrest or Sustained Ventricular Tachycardia in Patients with Hypertrophic Cardiomyopathy." *Journal of the American College of Cardiology* 33 (6): 1596‑1601.

Elliott, Perry, Juan Gimeno, Maite Tomé, et William McKenna. 2006. "Left Ventricular Outflow Tract Obstruction and Sudden Death in Hypertrophic Cardiomyopathy." *European Heart Journal* 27 (24): 3073; author reply 3073-3074. doi:10.1093/eurheartj/ehl383.

EXpert Group on Biomarkers. 2014. "Biomarkers in Cardiology--Part 1--in Heart Failure and Specific Cardiomyopathies." *Arquivos Brasileiros De Cardiologia* 103 (6): 451‑59. doi:10.5935/abc.20140184.

Femenía, Francisco, Maurico Arce, Jorge Van Grieken, Emilce Trucco, Luis Mont, Mauricio Abello, José L. Merino, et al. 2013. "Fragmented QRS as a Predictor of Arrhythmic Events in Patients with Hypertrophic Obstructive Cardiomyopathy." *Journal of Interventional Cardiac Electrophysiology: An International Journal of Arrhythmias and Pacing* 38 (3): 159‑65. doi:10.1007/s10840-013-9829-z.

Fernández, Adrián, Alejandro Quiroga, Juan Pablo Ochoa, Mauricio Mysuta, José Horacio Casabé, Marcelo Biagetti, Eduardo Guevara, Liliana E. Favaloro, Agostina M. Fava, et Néstor Galizio. 2016. "Validation of the 2014 European Society of Cardiology Sudden Cardiac Death Risk Prediction Model in Hypertrophic Cardiomyopathy in a Reference Center in South America." *The American Journal of Cardiology* 118 (1): 121‑26. doi:10.1016/ j.amjcard.2016.04.021.

Finocchiaro, Gherardo, Francois Haddad, Joshua W. Knowles, Colleen Caleshu, Aleksandra Pavlovic, Julian Homburger, Yael Shmargad, et al. 2015. "Cardiopulmonary Responses and Prognosis in Hypertrophic Cardiomyopathy: A Potential Role for Comprehensive Noninvasive Hemodynamic Assessment." *JACC. Heart Failure* 3 (5): 408‑18. doi:10.1016/j.jchf.2014.11.011.

Fraiche, Ariane, et Andrew Wang. 2016. "Hypertrophic Cardiomyopathy: New Evidence Since the 2011 American Cardiology of Cardiology Foundation and American Heart Association Guideline." *Current Cardiology Reports* 18 (8): 70. doi:10.1007/s11886-016-0751-8.

Francia, Pietro, Daria Santini, Beatrice Musumeci, Lorenzo Semprini, Carmen Adduci, Erika Pagannone, Giulia Proietti, Massimo Volpe, et Camillo Autore. 2014. "Clinical Impact of Nonsustained Ventricular Tachycardia Recorded by the Implantable Cardioverter-Defibrillator in Patients with Hypertrophic Cardiomyopathy." *Journal of Cardiovascular Electrophysiology* 25 (11): 1180‑87. doi:10.1111/jce.12492.

Frenneaux, M. P., P. J. Counihan, A. L. Caforio, T. Chikamori, et W. J. McKenna. 1990. "Abnormal Blood Pressure Response during Exercise in Hypertrophic Cardiomyopathy." *Circulation* 82 (6): 1995‑2002.

Gersh, Bernard J., Barry J. Maron, Robert O. Bonow, Joseph A. Dearani, Michael A. Fifer, Mark S. Link, Srihari S. Naidu, et al. 2011. "2011 ACCF/AHA Guideline for the Diagnosis and Treatment of Hypertrophic Cardiomyopathy: A Report of the American College of Cardiology Foundation/American Heart Association Task Force on Practice Guidelines. Developed in Collaboration with the American Association for Thoracic Surgery, American Society of Echocardiography, American Society of Nuclear Cardiology, Heart Failure Society of America, Heart Rhythm Society, Society for Cardiovascular Angiography and Interventions, and Society of Thoracic Surgeons." *Journal of the American College of Cardiology* 58 (25): e212-260. doi:10.1016/j.jacc.2011.06.011.

Gimeno, Juan R., Maite Tomé-Esteban, Carla Lofiego, José Hurtado, Antonios Pantazis, Bryan Mist, Pier Lambiase, William J. McKenna, et Perry M. Elliott. 2009. "Exercise-Induced Ventricular Arrhythmias and Risk of Sudden Cardiac Death in Patients with Hypertrophic

Cardiomyopathy." *European Heart Journal* 30 (21): 2599‑2605. doi:10.1093/eurheartj/ehp327.

Green, John J., Jeffery S. Berger, Christopher M. Kramer, et Michael Salerno. 2012. "Prognostic Value of Late Gadolinium Enhancement in Clinical Outcomes for Hypertrophic Cardiomyopathy." *JACC. Cardiovascular Imaging* 5 (4): 370‑77. doi:10.1016/j.jcmg.2011.11.021.

Hanneman, Kate, Andrew M. Crean, Lynne Williams, Hadas Moshonov, Susan James, Laura Jiménez-Juan, Christiane Gruner, Patrick Sparrow, Harry Rakowski, et Elsie T. Nguyen. 2014. "Cardiac Magnetic Resonance Imaging Findings Predict Major Adverse Events in Apical Hypertrophic Cardiomyopathy." *Journal of Thoracic Imaging* 29 (6): 331‑39. doi:10.1097/RTI.0000000000000115.

Hardarson, T., C. S. De la Calzada, R. Curiel, et J. F. Goodwin. 1973. "Prognosis and Mortality of Hypertrophic Obstructive Cardiomyopathy." *Lancet (London, England)* 2 (7844): 1462‑67.

Harris, Kevin M., Paolo Spirito, Martin S. Maron, Andrey G. Zenovich, Francesco Formisano, John R. Lesser, Shannon Mackey-Bojack, Warren J. Manning, James E. Udelson, et Barry J. Maron. 2006. "Prevalence, Clinical Profile, and Significance of Left Ventricular Remodeling in the End-Stage Phase of Hypertrophic Cardiomyopathy." *Circulation* 114 (3): 216‑25. doi:10.1161/CIRCULATIONAHA.105.583500.

Hinojar, Rocio, José Luis Zamorano, Ariana Gonzalez Gómez, Maria Plaza Martin, Amparo Esteban, Luis Miguel Rincón, Juan Carlos Portugal, José Julio Jimenez Nácher, et Covadonga Fernández-Golfín. 2017. "ESC Sudden-Death Risk Model in Hypertrophic Cardiomyopathy: Incremental Value of Quantitative Contrast-Enhanced CMR in Intermediate-Risk Patients." *Clinical Cardiology*, juin. doi:10.1002/clc.22735.

Inada, Keiichi, Jens Seiler, Kurt C. Roberts-Thomson, Daniel Steven, Jonathan Rosman, Roy M. John, Piotr Sobieszczyk, William G. Stevenson, et Usha B. Tedrow. 2011. "Substrate Characterization and Catheter Ablation for Monomorphic Ventricular Tachycardia in

Patients with Apical Hypertrophic Cardiomyopathy." *Journal of Cardiovascular Electrophysiology* 22 (1): 41‑48. doi:10.1111/j.1540-8167.2010.01875.x.

Ingles, J., A. Doolan, C. Chiu, J. Seidman, C. Seidman, et C. Semsarian. 2005. "Compound and Double Mutations in Patients with Hypertrophic Cardiomyopathy: Implications for Genetic Testing and Counselling." *Journal of Medical Genetics* 42 (10): e59. doi:10.1136/jmg.2005.033886.

Ismail, Tevfik F., Andrew Jabbour, Ankur Gulati, Amy Mallorie, Sadaf Raza, Thomas E. Cowling, Bibek Das, et al. 2014. "Role of Late Gadolinium Enhancement Cardiovascular Magnetic Resonance in the Risk Stratification of Hypertrophic Cardiomyopathy." *Heart (British Cardiac Society)* 100 (23): 1851‑58. doi:10.1136/heartjnl-2013-305471.

Jensen, Morten K., Christian Prinz, Dieter Horstkotte, Frank van Buuren, Thomas Bitter, Lothar Faber, et Henning Bundgaard. 2013. "Alcohol Septal Ablation in Patients with Hypertrophic Obstructive Cardiomyopathy: Low Incidence of Sudden Cardiac Death and Reduced Risk Profile." *Heart (British Cardiac Society)* 99 (14): 1012‑17. doi:10.1136/heartjnl-2012-303339.

Jong, Sanne de, Toon A. B. van Veen, Harold V. M. van Rijen, et Jacques M. T. de Bakker. 2011. "Fibrosis and Cardiac Arrhythmias." *Journal of Cardiovascular Pharmacology* 57 (6): 630‑38. doi:10.1097/FJC. 0b013e318207a35f.

Kawashiri, Masa-aki, Kenshi Hayashi, Tetsuo Konno, Noboru Fujino, Hidekazu Ino, et Masakazu Yamagishi. 2014. "Current Perspectives in Genetic Cardiovascular Disorders: From Basic to Clinical Aspects." *Heart and Vessels* 29 (2): 129‑41. doi:10.1007/s00380-013-0391-5.

Konno, Tetsuo, Stephen Chang, Jonathan G. Seidman, et Christine E. Seidman. 2010. "Genetics of Hypertrophic Cardiomyopathy." *Current Opinion in Cardiology* 25 (3): 205‑9. doi:10.1097/HCO.0b013e 3283375698.

Konno, Tetsuo, Masami Shimizu, Hidekazu Ino, Toru Matsuyama, Masato Yamaguchi, Hidenobu Terai, Kenshi Hayashi, et al. 2003. "A Novel

Missense Mutation in the Myosin Binding Protein-C Gene Is Responsible for Hypertrophic Cardiomyopathy with Left Ventricular Dysfunction and Dilation in Elderly Patients." *Journal of the American College of Cardiology* 41 (5): 781‐86.

Konstantinou, Dimitrios M., Georgios K. Efthimiadis, Vassilios Vassilikos, Stylianos Paraskevaidis, Efstathios Pagourelias, Barry J. Maron, et Haralambos Karvounis. 2016. "Implantable Cardioverter Defibrillators for Primary Prevention of Sudden Death in Hypertrophic Cardiomyopathy." *Journal of Cardiovascular Medicine (Hagerstown, Md.)* 17 (6): 433‐39. doi:10.2459/JCM.0000000000000333.

Kwon, Deborah H., Randolph M. Setser, Zoran B. Popović, Maran Thamilarasan, Srikanth Sola, Paul Schoenhagen, Mario J. Garcia, Scott D. Flamm, Harry M. Lever, et Milind Y. Desai. 2008. "Association of Myocardial Fibrosis, Electrocardiography and Ventricular Tachyarrhythmia in Hypertrophic Cardiomyopathy: A Delayed Contrast Enhanced MRI Study." *The International Journal of Cardiovascular Imaging* 24 (6): 617‐25. doi:10.1007/s10554-008-9292-6.

Lipshultz, Steven E., Lynn A. Sleeper, Jeffrey A. Towbin, April M. Lowe, E. John Orav, Gerald F. Cox, Paul R. Lurie, et al. 2003. "The Incidence of Pediatric Cardiomyopathy in Two Regions of the United States." *The New England Journal of Medicine* 348 (17): 1647‐55. doi:10.1056/NEJMoa021715.

Magrì, Damiano, Giuseppe Limongelli, Federica Re, Piergiuseppe Agostoni, Elisabetta Zachara, Michele Correale, Vittoria Mastromarino, et al. 2016. "Cardiopulmonary Exercise Test and Sudden Cardiac Death Risk in Hypertrophic Cardiomyopathy." *Heart (British Cardiac Society)* 102 (8): 602‐9. doi:10.1136/heartjnl-2015-308453.

Maki, S., H. Ikeda, A. Muro, N. Yoshida, A. Shibata, Y. Koga, et T. Imaizumi. 1998. "Predictors of Sudden Cardiac Death in Hypertrophic Cardiomyopathy." *The American Journal of Cardiology* 82 (6): 774‐78.

Maro, E. E., M. Janabi, et R. Kaushik. 2006. "Clinical and Echocardiographic Study of Hypertrophic Cardiomyopathy in Tanzania." *Tropical Doctor* 36 (4): 225‑27. doi:10.1258/004947506778604904.

Maron, B. J., J. M. Gardin, J. M. Flack, S. S. Gidding, T. T. Kurosaki, et D. E. Bild. 1995. "Prevalence of Hypertrophic Cardiomyopathy in a General Population of Young Adults. Echocardiographic Analysis of 4111 Subjects in the CARDIA Study. Coronary Artery Risk Development in (Young) Adults." *Circulation* 92 (4): 785‑89.

Maron, B. J., R. Mathenge, S. A. Casey, L. C. Poliac, et T. F. Longe. 1999. "Clinical Profile of Hypertrophic Cardiomyopathy Identified de Novo in Rural Communities." *Journal of the American College of Cardiology* 33 (6): 1590‑95.

Maron, B. J., I. Olivotto, P. Spirito, S. A. Casey, P. Bellone, T. E. Gohman, K. J. Graham, D. A. Burton, et F. Cecchi. 2000. "Epidemiology of Hypertrophic Cardiomyopathy-Related Death: Revisited in a Large Non-Referral-Based Patient Population." *Circulation* 102 (8): 858‑64.

Maron, B. J., W. C. Roberts, et S. E. Epstein. 1982. "Sudden Death in Hypertrophic Cardiomyopathy: A Profile of 78 Patients." *Circulation* 65 (7): 1388‑94.

Maron, Barry J., Susan A. Casey, Raymond H. Chan, Ross F. Garberich, Ethan J. Rowin, et Martin S. Maron. 2015. "Independent Assessment of the European Society of Cardiology Sudden Death Risk Model for Hypertrophic Cardiomyopathy." *The American Journal of Cardiology* 116 (5): 757‑64. doi:10.1016/j.amjcard.2015.05.047.

Maron, Barry J., Tammy S. Haas, Kevin M. Shannon, Adrian K. Almquist, et James S. Hodges. 2009. "Long-Term Survival after Cardiac Arrest in Hypertrophic Cardiomyopathy." *Heart Rhythm* 6 (7): 993‑97. doi:10.1016/j.hrthm.2009.03.014.

Maron, Barry J., Martin S. Maron, et Christopher Semsarian. 2012. "Double or Compound Sarcomere Mutations in Hypertrophic Cardiomyopathy: A Potential Link to Sudden Death in the Absence of Conventional Risk Factors." *Heart Rhythm* 9 (1): 57‑63. doi:10.1016/j.hrthm.2011.08.009.

Maron, Barry J., William J. McKenna, Gordon K. Danielson, Lukas J. Kappenberger, Horst J. Kuhn, Christine E. Seidman, Pravin M. Shah, et al. 2003. "American College of Cardiology/European Society of Cardiology Clinical Expert Consensus Document on Hypertrophic Cardiomyopathy. A Report of the American College of Cardiology Foundation Task Force on Clinical Expert Consensus Documents and the European Society of Cardiology Committee for Practice Guidelines." *Journal of the American College of Cardiology* 42 (9): 1687‑1713.

Maron, Barry J., Steve R. Ommen, Christopher Semsarian, Paolo Spirito, Iacopo Olivotto, et Martin S. Maron. 2014. "Hypertrophic Cardiomyopathy: Present and Future, with Translation into Contemporary Cardiovascular Medicine." *Journal of the American College of Cardiology* 64 (1): 83‑99. doi:10.1016/j.jacc.2014.05.003.

Maron, Barry J., Ethan J. Rowin, Susan A. Casey, Tammy S. Haas, Raymond H. M. Chan, James E. Udelson, Ross F. Garberich, et al. 2013. "Risk Stratification and Outcome of Patients with Hypertrophic Cardiomyopathy >=60 Years of Age." *Circulation* 127 (5): 585‑93. doi:10.1161/CIRCULATIONAHA.112.136085.

Maron, Barry J., Ethan J. Rowin, Susan A. Casey, Mark S. Link, John R. Lesser, Raymond H. M. Chan, Ross F. Garberich, James E. Udelson, et Martin S. Maron. 2015. "Hypertrophic Cardiomyopathy in Adulthood Associated With Low Cardiovascular Mortality With Contemporary Management Strategies." *Journal of the American College of Cardiology* 65 (18): 1915‑28. doi:10.1016/j.jacc.2015.02.061.

Maron, Barry J., Paolo Spirito, Mary J. Roman, Mary Paranicas, Peter M. Okin, Lyle G. Best, Elisa T. Lee, et Richard B. Devereux. 2004. "Prevalence of Hypertrophic Cardiomyopathy in a Population-Based Sample of American Indians Aged 51 to 77 Years (the Strong Heart Study)." *The American Journal of Cardiology* 93 (12): 1510‑14. doi:10.1016/j.amjcard.2004.03.007.

Maron, Barry J., Paolo Spirito, Win-Kuang Shen, Tammy S. Haas, Francesco Formisano, Mark S. Link, Andrew E. Epstein, et al. 2007. "Implantable Cardioverter-Defibrillators and Prevention of Sudden

Cardiac Death in Hypertrophic Cardiomyopathy." *JAMA* 298 (4): 405‑12. doi:10.1001/jama.298.4.405.

Maron, Martin S., Evan Appelbaum, Caitlin J. Harrigan, Jacki Buros, C. Michael Gibson, Connie Hanna, John R. Lesser, James E. Udelson, Warren J. Manning, et Barry J. Maron. 2008. "Clinical Profile and Significance of Delayed Enhancement in Hypertrophic Cardiomyopathy." *Circulation. Heart Failure* 1 (3): 184‑91. doi:10.1161/CIRCHEARTFAILURE.108.768119.

Maron, Martin S., John J. Finley, J. Martijn Bos, Thomas H. Hauser, Warren J. Manning, Tammy S. Haas, John R. Lesser, James E. Udelson, Michael J. Ackerman, et Barry J. Maron. 2008. "Prevalence, Clinical Significance, and Natural History of Left Ventricular Apical Aneurysms in Hypertrophic Cardiomyopathy." *Circulation* 118 (15): 1541‑49. doi:10.1161/CIRCULATIONAHA.108.781401.

Masri, Ahmad, Lee M. Pierson, Nicholas G. Smedira, Shikhar Agarwal, Bruce W. Lytle, Peyman Naji, Maran Thamilarasan, Harry M. Lever, Leslie S. Cho, et Milind Y. Desai. 2015. "Predictors of Long-Term Outcomes in Patients with Hypertrophic Cardiomyopathy Undergoing Cardiopulmonary Stress Testing and Echocardiography." *American Heart Journal* 169 (5): 684‑692.e1. doi:10.1016/j.ahj.2015.02.006.

Monserrat, Lorenzo, Perry M. Elliott, Juan R. Gimeno, Sanjay Sharma, Manuel Penas-Lado, et William J. McKenna. 2003. "Non-Sustained Ventricular Tachycardia in Hypertrophic Cardiomyopathy: An Independent Marker of Sudden Death Risk in Young Patients." *Journal of the American College of Cardiology* 42 (5): 873‑79.

Moon, James C. C., Emma Reed, Mary N. Sheppard, Andrew G. Elkington, Siew Yen Ho, Margaret Burke, Mario Petrou, et Dudley J. Pennell. 2004. "The Histologic Basis of Late Gadolinium Enhancement Cardiovascular Magnetic Resonance in Hypertrophic Cardiomyopathy." *Journal of the American College of Cardiology* 43 (12): 2260‑64. doi:10.1016/j.jacc.2004.03.035.

Moravsky, Gil, Efrat Ofek, Harry Rakowski, Jagdish Butany, Lynne Williams, Anthony Ralph-Edwards, Bernd J. Wintersperger, et Andrew Crean. 2013. "Myocardial Fibrosis in Hypertrophic

Cardiomyopathy: Accurate Reflection of Histopathological Findings by CMR." *JACC. Cardiovascular Imaging* 6 (5): 587‑96. doi:10.1016/j.jcmg.2012.09.018.

Morita, Norishige, William J. Mandel, Yoshinori Kobayashi, et Hrayr S. Karagueuzian. 2014. "Cardiac Fibrosis as a Determinant of Ventricular Tachyarrhythmias." *Journal of Arrhythmia* 30 (6): 389‑94. doi:10.1016/j.joa.2013.12.008.

Münch, Julia, Maxim Avanesov, Peter Bannas, Dennis Säring, Elisabeth Krämer, Giulia Mearini, Lucie Carrier, Anna Suling, Gunnar Lund, et Monica Patten. 2016. "Serum Matrix Metalloproteinases as Quantitative Biomarkers for Myocardial Fibrosis and Sudden Cardiac Death Risk Stratification in Patients with Hypertrophic Cardiomyopathy." *Journal of Cardiac Failure* 22 (10): 845‑50. doi:10.1016/j.cardfail.2016.03.010.

Ng, Choon Ta, Tek Siong Chee, Lee Fong Ling, Yian Ping Lee, Chi Keong Ching, Terrance S. J. Chua, Christopher Cheok, et Hean Yee Ong. 2011. "Prevalence of Hypertrophic Cardiomyopathy on an Electrocardiogram-Based Pre-Participation Screening Programme in a Young Male South-East Asian Population: Results from the Singapore Armed Forces Electrocardiogram and Echocardiogram Screening Protocol." *Europace: European Pacing, Arrhythmias, and Cardiac Electrophysiology: Journal of the Working Groups on Cardiac Pacing, Arrhythmias, and Cardiac Cellular Electrophysiology of the European Society of Cardiology* 13 (6): 883‑88. doi:10.1093/europace/eur051.

Nguyen, Thao P., Zhilin Qu, et James N. Weiss. 2014. "Cardiac Fibrosis and Arrhythmogenesis: The Road to Repair Is Paved with Perils." *Journal of Molecular and Cellular Cardiology* 70 (mai): 83‑91. doi:10.1016/j.yjmcc.2013.10.018.

Nugent, Alan W., Piers E. F. Daubeney, Patty Chondros, John B. Carlin, Steven D. Colan, Michael Cheung, Andrew M. Davis, C. W. Chow, Robert G. Weintraub, et National Australian Childhood Cardiomyopathy Study. 2005. "Clinical Features and Outcomes of Childhood Hypertrophic Cardiomyopathy: Results from a National

Population-Based Study." *Circulation* 112 (9): 1332‐38. doi:10.1161/CIRCULATIONAHA.104.530303.

Olivotto, I., B. J. Maron, A. Montereggi, F. Mazzuoli, A. Dolara, et F. Cecchi. 1999. "Prognostic Value of Systemic Blood Pressure Response during Exercise in a Community-Based Patient Population with Hypertrophic Cardiomyopathy." *Journal of the American College of Cardiology* 33 (7): 2044‐51.

Olivotto, Iacopo, Franco Cecchi, Corrado Poggesi, et Magdi H. Yacoub. 2012. "Patterns of Disease Progression in Hypertrophic Cardiomyopathy: An Individualized Approach to Clinical Staging." *Circulation. Heart Failure* 5 (4): 535‐46. doi:10.1161/CIRCHEART FAILURE.112.967026.

Olivotto, Iacopo, Francesca Girolami, Roberto Sciagrà, Michael J. Ackerman, Barbara Sotgia, J. Martijn Bos, Stefano Nistri, et al. 2011. "Microvascular Function Is Selectively Impaired in Patients with Hypertrophic Cardiomyopathy and Sarcomere Myofilament Gene Mutations." *Journal of the American College of Cardiology* 58 (8): 839‐48. doi:10.1016/j.jacc.2011.05.018.

Olivotto, Iacopo, Barry J. Maron, Evan Appelbaum, Caitlin J. Harrigan, Carol Salton, C. Michael Gibson, James E. Udelson, et al. 2010. "Spectrum and Clinical Significance of Systolic Function and Myocardial Fibrosis Assessed by Cardiovascular Magnetic Resonance in Hypertrophic Cardiomyopathy." *The American Journal of Cardiology* 106 (2): 261‐67. doi:10.1016/j.amjcard.2010.03.020.

Olivotto, Iacopo, Martin S. Maron, A. Selcuk Adabag, Susan A. Casey, Daniela Vargiu, Mark S. Link, James E. Udelson, Franco Cecchi, et Barry J. Maron. 2005. "Gender-Related Differences in the Clinical Presentation and Outcome of Hypertrophic Cardiomyopathy." *Journal of the American College of Cardiology* 46 (3): 480‐87. doi:10.1016/j.jacc.2005.04.043.

O'Mahony, Constantinos, Fatima Jichi, Menelaos Pavlou, Lorenzo Monserrat, Aristides Anastasakis, Claudio Rapezzi, Elena Biagini, et al. 2014. "A Novel Clinical Risk Prediction Model for Sudden Cardiac

Death in Hypertrophic Cardiomyopathy (HCM Risk-SCD).” *European Heart Journal* 35 (30): 2010‐20. doi:10.1093/eurheartj/eht439.

O’Mahony, Constantinos, Maite Tome-Esteban, Pier D. Lambiase, Antonios Pantazis, Shaughan Dickie, William J. McKenna, et Perry M. Elliott. 2013. “A Validation Study of the 2003 American College of Cardiology/European Society of Cardiology and 2011 American College of Cardiology Foundation/American Heart Association Risk Stratification and Treatment Algorithms for Sudden Cardiac Death in Patients with Hypertrophic Cardiomyopathy.” *Heart (British Cardiac Society)* 99 (8): 534‐41. doi:10.1136/heartjnl-2012-303271.

Ommen, Steve R., Barry J. Maron, Iacopo Olivotto, Martin S. Maron, Franco Cecchi, Sandro Betocchi, Bernard J. Gersh, et al. 2005. “Long-Term Effects of Surgical Septal Myectomy on Survival in Patients with Obstructive Hypertrophic Cardiomyopathy.” *Journal of the American College of Cardiology* 46 (3): 470‐76. doi:10.1016/j.jacc.2005.02.090.

Ozyilmaz, Sinem, Ozgur Akgul, Huseyin Uyarel, Hamdi Pusuroglu, Mehmet Gul, Muhammet Hulusi Satilmisoglu, Ismail Bolat, et al. 2017. “The Importance of the Neutrophil-to-Lymphocyte Ratio in Patients with Hypertrophic Cardiomyopathy.” *Revista Portuguesa De Cardiologia: Orgao Oficial Da Sociedade Portuguesa De Cardiologia = Portuguese Journal of Cardiology: An Official Journal of the Portuguese Society of Cardiology* 36 (4): 239‐46. doi:10.1016/j.repc.2016.09.014.

Rowin, Ethan J., et Martin S. Maron. 2016. “The Role of Cardiac MRI in the Diagnosis and Risk Stratification of Hypertrophic Cardiomyopathy.” *Arrhythmia & Electrophysiology Review* 5 (3): 197‐202. doi:10.15420/aer.2016:13:3.

Rubinshtein, Ronen, James F. Glockner, Steve R. Ommen, Philip A. Araoz, Michael J. Ackerman, Paul Sorajja, J. Martijn Bos, et al. 2010. “Characteristics and Clinical Significance of Late Gadolinium Enhancement by Contrast-Enhanced Magnetic Resonance Imaging in Patients with Hypertrophic Cardiomyopathy.” *Circulation. Heart*

Failure 3 (1): 51‑58. doi:10.1161/CIRCHEARTFAILURE.109.854026.

Sadoul, N., K. Prasad, P. M. Elliott, S. Bannerjee, M. P. Frenneaux, et W. J. McKenna. 1997. "Prospective Prognostic Assessment of Blood Pressure Response during Exercise in Patients with Hypertrophic Cardiomyopathy." *Circulation* 96 (9): 2987‑91.

Sakamoto, Naka, Yuichiro Kawamura, Nobuyuki Sato, Asami Nimura, Motoki Matsuki, Atsushi Yamauchi, Takayasu Kanno, et al. 2015. "Late Gadolinium Enhancement on Cardiac Magnetic Resonance Represents the Depolarizing and Repolarizing Electrically Damaged Foci Causing Malignant Ventricular Arrhythmia in Hypertrophic Cardiomyopathy." *Heart Rhythm* 12 (6): 1276‑84. doi:10.1016/j.hrthm.2015.02.004.

Sakamoto, T., C. Tei, M. Murayama, H. Ichiyasu, et Y. Hada. 1976. "Giant T Wave Inversion as a Manifestation of Asymmetrical Apical Hypertrophy (AAH) of the Left Ventricle. Echocardiographic and Ultrasono-Cardiotomographic Study." *Japanese Heart Journal* 17 (5): 611‑29.

Schinkel, Arend F. L., Pieter A. Vriesendorp, Eric J. G. Sijbrands, Luc J. L. M. Jordaens, Folkert J. ten Cate, et Michelle Michels. 2012. "Outcome and Complications after Implantable Cardioverter Defibrillator Therapy in Hypertrophic Cardiomyopathy: Systematic Review and Meta-Analysis." *Circulation. Heart Failure* 5 (5): 552‑59. doi:10.1161/CIRCHEARTFAILURE.112.969626.

Spirito, P., P. Bellone, K. M. Harris, P. Bernabo, P. Bruzzi, et B. J. Maron. 2000. "Magnitude of Left Ventricular Hypertrophy and Risk of Sudden Death in Hypertrophic Cardiomyopathy." *The New England Journal of Medicine* 342 (24): 1778‑85. doi:10.1056/NEJM200006153422403.

Spirito, P., C. Rapezzi, C. Autore, P. Bruzzi, P. Bellone, P. Ortolani, P. V. Fragola, F. Chiarella, M. Zoni-Berisso, et A. Branzi. 1994. "Prognosis of Asymptomatic Patients with Hypertrophic Cardiomyopathy and Nonsustained Ventricular Tachycardia." *Circulation* 90 (6): 2743‑47.

Spirito, Paolo, Camillo Autore, Claudio Rapezzi, Paola Bernabò, Roberto Badagliacca, Martin S. Maron, Sergio Bongioanni, et al. 2009.

"Syncope and Risk of Sudden Death in Hypertrophic Cardiomyopathy." *Circulation* 119 (13): 1703‑10. doi:10.1161/CIRCULATIONAHA.108.798314.

Stroumpoulis, Konstantinos I., Ioannis N. Pantazopoulos, et Theodoros T. Xanthos. 2010. "Hypertrophic Cardiomyopathy and Sudden Cardiac Death." *World Journal of Cardiology* 2 (9): 289‑98. doi:10.4330/wjc.v2.i9.289.

Sugrue, Alan, Ammar M. Killu, Christopher V. DeSimone, Anwar A. Chahal, Josh C. Vogt, Vaclav Kremen, JoJo Hai, et al. 2017. "Utility of T-Wave Amplitude as a Non-Invasive Risk Marker of Sudden Cardiac Death in Hypertrophic Cardiomyopathy." *Open Heart* 4 (1): e000561. doi:10.1136/openhrt-2016-000561.

Trivedi, Amar, et Bradley P. Knight. 2016. "ICD Therapy for Primary Prevention in Hypertrophic Cardiomyopathy." *Arrhythmia & Electrophysiology Review* 5 (3): 188‑96. doi:10.15420/aer.2016:30:2.

Van Driest, S. L., B. J. Maron, et M. J. Ackerman. 2004. "From Malignant Mutations to Malignant Domains: The Continuing Search for Prognostic Significance in the Mutant Genes Causing Hypertrophic Cardiomyopathy." *Heart (British Cardiac Society)* 90 (1): 7‑8.

Varnava, A. M., P. M. Elliott, N. Mahon, M. J. Davies, et W. J. McKenna. 2001. "Relation between Myocyte Disarray and Outcome in Hypertrophic Cardiomyopathy." *The American Journal of Cardiology* 88 (3): 275‑79.

Veselka, Josef, Nandan S. Anavekar, et Philippe Charron. 2017. "Hypertrophic Obstructive Cardiomyopathy." *Lancet (London, England)* 389 (10075): 1253‑67. doi:10.1016/S0140-6736(16)31321-6.

Veselka, Josef, Pavol Tomašov, et David Zemánek. 2011. "Long-Term Effects of Varying Alcohol Dosing in Percutaneous Septal Ablation for Obstructive Hypertrophic Cardiomyopathy: A Randomized Study with a Follow-up up to 11 Years." *The Canadian Journal of Cardiology* 27 (6): 763‑67. doi:10.1016/j.cjca.2011.09.001.

Viswanathan, Karthik, Adrian M. Suszko, Moloy Das, Nicholas Jackson, Michael Gollob, Douglas Cameron, Danna Spears, et al. 2016. "Rapid

Device-Detected Nonsustained Ventricular Tachycardia in the Risk Stratification of Hypertrophic Cardiomyopathy." *Pacing and Clinical Electrophysiology: PACE* 39 (7): 642‑51. doi:10.1111/pace.12861.

Vriesendorp, Pieter A., Arend F. L. Schinkel, Max Liebregts, Dominic A. M. J. Theuns, Johan van Cleemput, Folkert J. Ten Cate, Rik Willems, et Michelle Michels. 2015. "Validation of the 2014 European Society of Cardiology Guidelines Risk Prediction Model for the Primary Prevention of Sudden Cardiac Death in Hypertrophic Cardiomyopathy." *Circulation. Arrhythmia and Electrophysiology* 8 (4): 829‑35. doi:10.1161/CIRCEP.114.002553.

Wang, Jizheng, Yilu Wang, Yubao Zou, Kai Sun, Zhimin Wang, Hu Ding, Jinqing Yuan, et al. 2014. "Malignant Effects of Multiple Rare Variants in Sarcomere Genes on the Prognosis of Patients with Hypertrophic Cardiomyopathy." *European Journal of Heart Failure* 16 (9): 950‑57. doi:10.1002/ejhf.144.

Watkins, H., W. J. McKenna, L. Thierfelder, H. J. Suk, R. Anan, A. O'Donoghue, P. Spirito, A. Matsumori, C. S. Moravec, et J. G. Seidman. 1995. "Mutations in the Genes for Cardiac Troponin T and Alpha-Tropomyosin in Hypertrophic Cardiomyopathy." *The New England Journal of Medicine* 332 (16): 1058‑64. doi:10.1056/NEJM199504203321603.

Weissler-Snir, Adaya, Arnon Adler, Lynne Williams, Christiane Gruner, et Harry Rakowski. 2017. "Prevention of Sudden Death in Hypertrophic Cardiomyopathy: Bridging the Gaps in Knowledge." *European Heart Journal* 38 (22): 1728‑37. doi:10.1093/eurheartj/ehw268.

Weng, Zhen, Jialu Yao, Raymond H. Chan, Jun He, Xiangjun Yang, Yafeng Zhou, et Yang He. 2016. "Prognostic Value of LGE-CMR in HCM: A Meta-Analysis." *JACC. Cardiovascular Imaging* 9 (12): 1392‑1402. doi:10.1016/j.jcmg.2016.02.031.

Werf, Christian van der, Irene M. van Langen, et Arthur A. M. Wilde. 2010. "Sudden Death in the Young: What Do We Know about It and How to Prevent?" *Circulation. Arrhythmia and Electrophysiology* 3 (1): 96‑104. doi:10.1161/CIRCEP.109.877142.

Wilkoff, Bruce L., Laurent Fauchier, Martin K. Stiles, Carlos A. Morillo, Sana M. Al-Khatib, Jesús Almendral, Luis Aguinaga, et al. 2016. "2015 HRS/EHRA/APHRS/SOLAECE Expert Consensus Statement on Optimal Implantable Cardioverter-Defibrillator Programming and Testing." *Heart Rhythm* 13 (2): e50-86. doi:10.1016/j.hrthm.2015.11.018.

Zhu, S. H., Y. Li, W. Huang, H. Jiang, S. N. Li, L. Chen, S. Huang, H. S. Yu, et B. Xu. 2017. "(Feasibility of the 2014 European guidelines risk prediction model for sudden cardiac death in hypertrophic cardiomyopathy in Chinese patients)." *Zhonghua Xin Xue Guan Bing Za Zhi* 45 (5): 404‑8.

Zou, Yubao, Lei Song, Zhimin Wang, Aiqun Ma, Tangwei Liu, Huimin Gu, Sailan Lu, et al. 2004. "Prevalence of Idiopathic Hypertrophic Cardiomyopathy in China: A Population-Based Echocardiographic Analysis of 8080 Adults." *The American Journal of Medicine* 116 (1): 14‑18.

In: Hypertrophic Cardiomyopathy
Editor: Ikram Kammoun

ISBN: 978-1-53613-003-4

Chapter 7

CATHETER-BASED TECHNIQUES FOR SEPTAL REDUCTION IN OBSTRUCTIVE HYPERTROPHIC CARDIOMYOPATHY

Marouane Boukhris[1,*], Salvatore D Tomasello[2], Alfredo R Galassi[3] and Salem Kachboura[4]

[1]Department of cardiology, Tunis ElManar University, Ariana, Tunisia
[2]Cardiology Division, Cannizzaro Hospital, Catania, Italy
[3]Department of Clinical and Experimental Medicine, University of Catania, Catania, Italy
Department of Cardiology, University Heart Center, Zurich, Switzerland
[4]Department of cardiology, Tunis ElManar University, Ariana, Tunisia

ABSTRACT

Hypertrophic cardiomyopathy (HCM) is the most common inheritable cardiac disease, present in 1 in 500 of the general population. Roughly one-third of patients with HCM have physiology consistent with resting left ventricular outflow tract obstruction (LVOTO), another third

* Corresponding author: mar1bou@hotmail.com.

have obstruction elicited only by provocative maneuvers, and the remaining third are fully non obstructive. LVOTO is associated with higher morbidity and mortality in patients with HCM. Septal myectomy is considered to be the "gold standard" for treating severe obstructive HCM. Since 1994, alcohol septal ablation (ASA) has been performed widely and successfully, with short- and intermediate-term clinical outcome. In addition, other interventional techniques for septal reduction in case of obstructive HCM have been explored.

Keywords: obstructive hypertrophic cardiomyopathy, left ventricular outflow tract obstruction, myectomy, septal reduction, alcohol septal ablation

Introduction

Hypertrophic cardiomyopathy (HCM) is the most common inheritable cardiac disease, present in 1 in 500 of the general population (B. J. Maron et al. 1995). Roughly one-third of patients with HCM have physiology consistent with resting left ventricular outflow tract obstruction (LVOTO), another third have obstruction elicited only by provocative maneuvers, and the remaining third are fully non obstructive (M. S. Maron et al. 2006). LVOTO in HCM is usually the combination of basal septal hypertrophy and systolic anterior motion (SAM) of the mitral valve. A gradient of >50 mmHg is usually considered to be the threshold at which LVOT obstruction becomes hemodynamically significant (Gersh et al. 2011; Authors/Task Force members et al. 2014). LVOTO is associated with higher morbidity and mortality in patients with HCM [B. J. Maron et al. 1995; M. S. Maron et al. 2006]. Surgical septal myectomy has been considered to be the "gold standard" for treating severe obstructive HCM (B. J. Maron 2007).

First performed by Cleland in 1958, surgical myectomy was the first invasive treatment for obstructive HCM (Goodwin et al. 1960). In1960, Morrow used a technique in which a small, rectangular bar of muscle from just below the aortic valve to beyond the site of mitral-septal contact was resected (Morrow et al. 1975). For the next four decades, ventricular septal myectomy was considered to be the "gold standard" for treating severe obstructive HCM, reducing LVOT gradients significantly in over 90% of cases, reducing SAM-related mitral regurgitation, and improving exercise capacity and symptoms (McCully et al. 1996;Khouzam and Naidu 2014).

Nonetheless, in real world practice, several subgroups of patients were poor candidates for surgery, particularly those with advanced age and significant comorbidity. Average age at myectomy in all series has been~ 40 years, a population typically at low-risk for surgical morbidity and mortality (Khouzam and Naidu 2014). This young average age implies that symptomatic older patients with comorbidities have historically been excluded.

With the development of interventional cardiology, the concept of less invasive treatment of LVOTO has become more and more attractive. In 1994, two groups of investigators almost simultaneously developed the alcohol septal ablation (ASA) for the treatment of obstructive HCM. Gietzen presented their preliminary findings at the Annual Congress of the German Cardiac Society (in April), whereas Sigwart presented his results at the Royal Brompton Hospital in London (in June) publishing subsequently the first 3 cases in The Lancet (Sigwart 1995). Since that time, ASA has been performed widely and successfully, with short- and intermediate-term clinical outcome. Furthermore, other interventional techniques for septal reduction in case of obstructive HCM have been explored.

In the current chapter, we will describe the different catheter-based techniques for septal reduction available in the armamentarium of the interventional cardiologist when treating patients with obstructive HCM, evaluating their outcome according to reported data through literature.

Alcohol Septal Ablation

Indications and Guidelines

Table 1 summarizes the indications and contraindications of ASA.

Table 1. Indications and contraindications of ASA

INDICATIONS
Clinical characteristics
1. Severe symptoms (NYHA Class 3–4 heart failure, CCS Class 3–4 angina pectoris, or recurrent pre-syncope or syncope) despite optimal drug therapy
2. Mild or moderate symptoms but with recurrent presyncope, syncope, or clinical decompensation due to recurrent paroxysmal atrial fibrillation
3. Symptoms deemed to be primarily due to LVOTO or consequences of chronic LVOTO
4. Life expectancy >1 year, and absence of severe comorbidity limiting functional status or any improvement that would be achieved by relief of LVOTO (i.e., severe dementia, non-ambulatory patient)
Anatomic characteristics
1. Subaortic gradient of at least 50 mm Hg (at baseline or with provocation) despite optimal drug therapy
2. Subaortic obstruction due to SAM of the mitral valve leaflet or associated structures
3. One or more septal perforators likely to serve the target myocardium contributing to LVOTO.
4. Septum at region of obstruction is >15 mm thickness
CONTRAINDICATIONS
Anatomic characteristics
1. Gradient due to severe abnormalities of the mitral valve or associated valvular apparatus, or abnormal membranes in the outflow tract or above the valve (subvalvular or supravalvular or membranes).
2. Mid-ventricular obstruction due to severe concentric hypertrophy, with no contribution of mitral valve
3. Severe coronary disease that independently warrants coronary artery bypass grafting
4. Severe valvular aortic stenosis (or other valvular pathology) that would independently warrant surgical correction
5. Septal mass at region of obstruction >30 mm thickness

Abbreviations: ASA = Alcohol septal ablation; CCS = Canadian Cardiovascular Society; LVOTO = left ventricular outflow tract obstruction; NYHA = New York Heart Association; SAM = systolic anterior motion.

ASA is considered feasible when all of the following anatomic, hemodynamic, and clinical criteria are present. In addition to the listed indications for alcohol septal ablation, there are several factors that may suggest one invasive therapy as more preferential than the other. For example, factors favoring ASA include advanced age or significant comorbidities that would elevate surgical risk, a previously implanted pacemaker (PM) or internal cardioverter defibrillator (ICD) that reduces procedural risk, ideal anatomy for alcohol septal ablation (small, focal septal bulge and appropriate sized and placed septal perforator to the target myocardium), patients who have already had open-heart surgery (particularly prior failed myectomy), patients with prior stroke, and those with baseline right bundle branch block (RBBB), because of the high likelihood of PM requirement with surgical myectomy (Khouzam and Naidu 2014). Conversely, factors against ASA (favoring surgery) include young age (particularly pediatric patients and adolescents), considerable myocardial thickening >30 mm, mid-ventricular obstruction, intrinsic significant valvular disease, membrane, or significant coronary stenoses unamenable to angioplasty, and the presence of baseline left bundle branch block (LBBB) (Khouzam and Naidu 2014).

Moreover, patients who strongly prefer a minimally invasive approach and in whom anatomically both procedures are judged comparable by both operators may opt for ASA. More importantly, local and regional expertise in one or both procedures should be taken into consideration. ASA should only be performed by a specially trained interventional cardiologist. Guidelines for competency include both cognitive and technical skills, as well as appropriate staff training and volume (Gersh et al. 2011; Authors/Task Force members et al. 2014). Practically, the first 5 cases should be proctored, and operators may avail themselves of national training courses or sessions at professional society meetings to achieve some of these skills and abilities.

Thereafter, institutions should both continue performing at least 5–10 procedures per year and also continue to follow patients longitudinally as part of a multidisciplinary HCM program offering a full range of services and treatments, including surgical myectomy. Hence, surgeon training is vital to a successful and appropriate ASA program (Khouzam and Naidu 2014).

The 2011 ACCF/AHA Guidelines for the Diagnosis and Management of HCM, advocates for ASA as a good alternative to surgery in those with significant comorbidity or advanced age (Class 2a), and allows the procedure for those at lower surgical risk after a balanced discussion (Class 2b) (Gersh et al. 2011). In the 2014 ESC guidelines, no specific recommendations were assigned to ASA (Authors/Task Force members et al. 2014).

Procedural Details

Only minimal sedation is preferable as it could reduce or eliminate gradients in some patients. The procedure is performed through the radial or femoral approach and identification of the septal branch to be treated, as well as gradient measurements before and after ASA, are monitored by echocardiography. Two transducers are required: one transducing pressure from the left ventricular apex via a 5F pigtail catheter and the other transducing pressure from the 6F arterial sheath. Resting and provocable gradients are determined, confirming the sub-aortic location and dynamic nature. Slow pullback of an end-hole catheter across the outflow tract and aortic valve may be necessary. Generally, provocable gradients are observed during the strain phase of the Valsalva maneuver, on the post–premature ventricular complex beat, and with the latter maneuver during the strain phase of the Valsalva maneuver (combined maneuvers). A temporary PM should be inserted before the procedure, especially in patients with a high risk of post-procedural atrioventricular (AV) block. It should be mandatory in patients with previous left bundle branch block (LBBB).

JL4 is generally the preferred guide catheter because it might slightly reduce the risk of guide-related coronary dissection in comparison with XB or EBU guide catheters.

Careful angiogram analysis is capital to identify all potential septal arteries before settling on the one with the highest potential for initial success. Indeed, septal perforators could also originate from the ramus intermedius, the left main bifurcation, and the proximal right coronary artery. Typically, a 0.014” coronary guidewire is advanced to the presupposed septal branch. A short (6-8mm) over-the-wire balloon is then advanced into the septal branch and inflated at small pressure (6-8 atm). The guidewire is removed and a small amount of angiographic contrast (0.5 ml) injected into the septal branch to ensure no spill back into the parent artery or collateral connection to other septal or major epicardial vessels. Myocardial contrast echocardiography is then performed to demonstrate the area of myocardium supplied by the selected vessel. Once the target artery has been satisfactorily identified, a small volume (1-3 ml) of absolute alcohol (95-96°) is injected slowly (usually 1 ml/min), followed by a 0.3 cc saline flush. Balloon occlusion should be maintained for at least 3 to 5 minutes. During the procedure, multiple images angiograms should be performed to check the stability of the guide and balloon system, and the maintenance of normal flow in the left anterior descending must be assured throughout. A final angiographic image is taken to confirm the septal branch no-reflow and rule out any unwanted coronary artery damage. In case of failure, (gradient reduction <50% and area of ASA incomplete), a second septal branch may be explored during the same procedure. After ASA, the patient is kept under coronary care supervision in the intensive care unit for at least 48 hours. Indication for definitive PM is decided at day two or three to allow intrinsic conduction to recover in case of acute reversible AV block. Discharge is generally after 5 days if no complication has occurred. Table 2 underlines the 10 most important recommendations when performing ASA.

Table 2. Important recommendations when performing ASA

Recommendations
1. Check suitable septal anatomy on coronary angiography
2. Prefer radial access with minimal sedation
3. Consider temporary PM (especially if prior LBBB)
4. Guiding catheter in the left main after anticoagulation (prefer JL4)
5. Wiring and short OTW balloon in the targeted septal
6. Guidance by echography in the region supplied by the selected septal
7. Injection of an appropriate quantity of alcohol >94° (1 ml/mm of septal diameter)
8. Keep balloon inflated for 3-5 minutes after alcohol injection
9. Keep the patient monitored for 24-48 hours in ICU
10. Check efficacy by gradient reduction and CK/troponin peak

Abbreviations:

ASA = alcohol septal ablation; CK = creatine kinase; ICU = intensive care unit; LBBB = left bundle branch block; OTW = over-the-wire; PM = pacemaker.

Peri-Procedural Complications

The most common complication after ASA is the development of complete AV block, seen in up to half of patients within the first 24 hours; however, only 5–10% of patients ultimately will require permanent PM. Patients with first degree AV block and those with LBBB are at higher risk, justifying pre-procedure temporary PM placement in this subset of patients (Gimeno, Tomé, and McKenna 2012). It is also important to notice that the incidence of AV block has decreased since the use of myocardial contrast echocardiography, as well as by reducing the amount and speed of ethanol infusion (Cuisset and Lefèvre 2016).

Other complications are rarely reported such as coronary dissection and inadvertent ethanol leakage into a major coronary (<1% of patients), or perforation of the right ventricle due to the temporary PM (<2%) (14) (Table 3).

Table 3. Post-procedural complications following ASA

Post-procedural complications following ASA
1. Complete AV block
2. Coronary dissection
3. Myocardial infarction
4. Ventricular septal defect
5. Ventricular arrhythmias
6. Tamponade from PM implantation
7. Pericarditis
8. Bleeding complications
9. Complications of additional procedural (PM or ICD)

Abbreviations

ASA = Alcohol septal ablation; AV = atrioventricular; ICD = Implantable cardioverter defibrillator; PM = pacemaker.

Clinical Outcome (ASA vs. Surgical Myectomy)

In order to compare the two techniques, a randomized controlled trial should be performed to end the discussion about which procedure is best.

However, in the present setting, such a trial would require 1,200 patients eligible and willing to be randomized to ASA or surgery. Because the prevalence of HCM is 1 in 500 and <10% of these patients require ASA, such a trial is almost impossible to perform (Olivotto et al. 2007). Therefore, the only way to compare the two at the moment is by retrospective analysis.

Furthermore, in a meta-analysis, Liebregts and colleagues found only 6 studies comparing ASA with myectomy; whereas, 44 studies were found to focus on the outcomes of one of the 2 interventions (Liebregts et al. 2015). This finding could be interpreted as a sign of ongoing polarization towards these two techniques.

Peri-Procedural Complications and Immediate Outcome

After ASA, LVOT gradient shows a triphasic response. In the first phase, there is an immediate decrease in the gradient following the procedure. This has been attributed to the stunning of the septum. In the second phase, there might be some increase in the LVOTO because of peri-infarct edema. This stage lasts for 7–14 days after the procedure. In the third phase, the LVOTO gradually decreases, as the scar forms over weeks and months and the septum gradually becomes thinner (Lakkis et al. 2000; Yoerger et al. 2006).

In the meta-analysis by Liebregts (Liebregts et al. 2015), periprocedural mortality rate following myectomy was found to be twice as high as that with ASA. However, peri-procedural care was potentially less-developed at the time of the old studies. When studies prior to 2000 were excluded, the periprocedural mortality rates of both procedures were practically the same. For ventricular arrhythmias, meta-analysis found a similar incidence after both procedures. However, when only focusing on studies after 2000, the periprocedural event rate of ventricular arrhythmias was 2.2% after ASA as opposed to 0.6% after myectomy ($p = 0.055$). This latter fact is due to the increased arrhythmogenicity of an acute myocardial infarction.

The need for PM implantation after ASA or myectomy is variable between studies (0% to 22% in ASA cases, vs. 0% to 13% after myectomy) (Liebregts, Vriesendorp, and Ten Berg 2017). In their meta-analysis, Liebregts (Liebregts et al. 2015) reported 10% need for permanent PM following ASA procedures, while this rate was 4% following surgery.

On the other hand, myectomy was reported to lead to a slightly greater decrease in post-procedural LVOT gradient (Agarwal et al. 2010) whereas, no significant differences were observed in the reintervention rate immediately after the two procedures (Liebregts et al. 2015; Agarwal et al. 2010). However, long-term follow-up is required to better assess this outcome parameter.

Long-Term Outcome

Sorajja et al. (Sorajja et al. 2012) reviewed 601 patients with obstructive HCM who underwent invasive therapy (including 138 who underwent ASA). Patients who were referred to ASA represented a higher risk population based on baseline characteristics including age. Procedural complications were relatively high: death (1.4%), tamponade (3%), malignant arrhythmias (3%), and permanent PM implantation (20%). Conversely, the complication rate after surgical myectomy in an age- and gender-matched cohort was statistically lower at 5% ($p < 0.0001$). Nonetheless, survival at 4 years in the ASA group was 88%, which did not differ from surgery ($p = 0.18$). Survival or NYHA class 3 or 4 symptoms was 76.4% at 4 years, with 51% of patients asymptomatic. Interestingly, patients ≤65 years of age fared better with myectomy ($p = 0.01$). Similarly, in a cohort of 1,047 patients with HCM, Vriesendorp et al. (Vriesendorp et al. 2014) reported similar survival for ASA and myectomy after a mean follow-up period of 7.6 years; this survival was comparable to that of patients with nonobstructive HCM.

To compare the outcomes of ASA and myectomy, Ten Cate et al. (ten Cate et al. 2010) focused on the composite outcome cardiac death, aborted sudden cardiac death, and appropriate ICD shock. Patients who underwent ASA experienced 5-fold higher incidence in the estimated annual primary endpoint rate in comparison with those who underwent surgery (4.4% vs. 0.9%). No discrimination was made between early and late events in this study. When assessing the composite endpoint for the different ASA cohorts included in the meta-analysis (Liebregts et al. 2015), half of them showed estimated rates <0.9% per year.

The incidence of need for additional sepal reduction reintervention (either percutaneous or surgical) was 7.7% in ASA cases versus 1.6% following myectomy. Because of these reinterventions, none of the aforementioned studies observed a difference in symptoms as assessed by the New York Heart Association (NYHA) functional class at late follow-up between ASA-treated and myectomy-treated patients. Similarly in another study, when patients were explicitly asked using a questionnaire at late follow-up, no differences in functional status were noticed when comparing these two approaches (Steggerda et al. 2014).

Catheter-Based Techniques for Septal Ablation

Despite its efficiency in appropriately selected patients, ASA may be responsible for life-threatening complications such as conduction disturbances (particularly complete AV block), ventricular arrhythmias, and massive myocardial necrosis. Therefore, various alternative modalities have been tried as a substitute of alcohol such as coils (Lafont et al. 2005), microspheres, covered stents, n-butyl cyanoacrylate (glue) septal ablation (GSA) (Llamas-Esperón and Sandoval-Navarrete 2007) and radiofrequency ablation (T. Lawrenz and Kuhn 2004).

Glue Septal Ablation

GSA has been known to be an intravascular embolic agent in the treatment of vascular malformations and hemorrhage. Matos et al. (Matos et al. 2005) performed a feasibility study for the use of controlled myocardial infarction in experimental models (dogs). The investigators showed that GSA does not escape from the target artery through capillaries or small collateral vessels, hence producing a sharply limited scar confined to the supply zone of the injected vessel.

The main principles of the GSA procedure are similar to ASA. Reducing the interventricular septal thickness and dynamic LVOTO by embolizing the septal arterial branches via trans-catheter route is the main objective of GSA. Obviously, the indications of GSA are the same as those of ASA.

Okutucu et al. (Okutucu, Aytemir, and Oto 2016) reported the outcome of 27 patients with obstructive HCM who underwent GSA: 1 septal ablation (19 patients), 2 septal ablations (8 patients). Following GSA, peak LVOT gradient was reduced significantly (from 77.8 ± 18.0 to 20.5 ± 11.7mmHg; $p < 0.001$); this reduction persisted at 1-year follow-up. NYHA functional class improved (3.0 ± 0.3 vs. 1.5 ± 0.8; $p < 0.001$) and interventricular septum thickness decreased (18.4 ± 2.6 vs. 14.7 ± 1.9mm; $p < 0.001$) significantly at one year of follow-up. Only four (14.8%) patients had the peak LVOT gradient $\geq$50mmHg and two (7.4%) patients had NYHA class III symptoms.

Further larger studies are warranted to better evaluate the results of GSA in symptomatic patients with obstructive HCM, in comparison with ASA and myectomy.

Coil Embolization

A French registry assessing coil embolization was published with satisfactory results and a low rate of complications (Durand et al. 2008). In this study, Durand et al. reported the outcome of 20 patients with obstructive HCM who underwent successful septal embolization (in all cases) using coils. The investigators demonstrated a significant reduction of gradient with very low complications, except for one (5%) who experienced ventricular septum defect. However, the rich collateralization of the septum may challenge the possibility of effectively reducing long-term gradients by ischemia alone. In this pilot study, the gradient reduction was maintained at six months following the procedure, but no long-term data is available.

Endocardial Radiofrequency Ablation of Septal Hypertrophy (ERASH)

In patients not suitable for surgery and not amenable to ischemia-related septal ablation techniques, another approach by direct endocavitary ablation (essentially radiofrequency) has been proposed. Lawrenz et al. (Thorsten Lawrenz et al. 2011) performed ERASH in a cohort of 19 adults (eight of whom had already undergone unsuccessful ASA because of inappropriate coronary anatomy). Although a minor reduction in the magnitude of septal hypertrophy was found at follow up, deep scars were visible within the septum on cardiac magnetic resonance. Conversely, following ASA, a more marked change in septal thickness is typically observed during diastole. Nonetheless, an important decrease in resting and provoked gradients was observed as well as a significant improvement in dyspnea status after ERASH procedures. Lawrenz et al. (Thorsten Lawrenz et al. 2011) claimed that ERASH might represent a new efficient and therapeutic alternative in the treatment of obstructive HCM, providing a significant and sustained decrease in LVOTO as well as symptom improvement. This approach was relatively safe, although 4 (21%) patients experienced complete AV block and required PM implantation. It could be indicated in patients not amenable to ASA or myectomy.

Similarly to other ischemia-related septal ablation techniques, the most important step in the the ERASH procedure is the exact localization of the SAM-interventricular septum contact point (the target), generally performed by transesophageal or intracardiac echocardiography.

Data on short and long-term outcomes and complications of the ERASH procedure are scarcely reported throughout literature. In addition, because of the small sample size of the relevant literature (a total of 60 cases), it is difficult to appropriately evaluate this technique and clearly identify its indications. At this time, ERASH should only be considered for the patient for whom surgical myectomy is not suitable after an unsuccessful transcoronary ASA procedure. In the future, large-scale studies are needed to make the ERASH more widespread. Mapping the AV node and bundle bunch conduction sites may be an added effect to avoid conductance trouble following the ablation.

Conclusion

Surgical myectomy is still considered the gold standard for treating patients with obstructive HCM. Septal ablation via alcohol application is considered to be a reliable treatment alternative in well-selected patients. In expert hands, ASA is associated with a low rate of complications and good long-term outcome. Newer techniques like GSA and ERASH could provide further options in the armamentarium of the interventional cardiologist for specific subsets of patients with obstructive HCM.

References

Agarwal, Shikhar E., Murat, Tuzcu., Milind, Y. Desai., Nicholas, Smedira., Harry, M. Lever., Bruce, W. Lytle. & Samir, R. Kapadia. (2010). "Updated Meta-Analysis of Septal Alcohol Ablation versus Myectomy for Hypertrophic Cardiomyopathy." *Journal of the American College of Cardiology*, *55* (8), 823–34. doi:10.1016/j.jacc.2009.09.047.

Authors/Task Force members, Perry, M. Elliott., Aris, Anastasakis., Michael, A. Borger., Martin, Borggrefe., Franco, Cecchi., Philippe, Charron., et al. (2014). "2014 ESC Guidelines on Diagnosis and Management of Hypertrophic Cardiomyopathy: The Task Force for the Diagnosis and Management of Hypertrophic Cardiomyopathy of the European Society of Cardiology (ESC)." *European Heart Journal*, *35* (39), 2733–79. doi:10.1093/eurheartj/ehu284.

Cate, Folkert J. ten., Osama, I. I. Soliman., Michelle, Michels., Dominic, A. M. J. Theuns., Peter, L. de Jong., Marcel, L. Geleijnse. & Patrick, W. Serruys. (2010). "Long-Term Outcome of Alcohol Septal Ablation in Patients with Obstructive Hypertrophic Cardiomyopathy: A Word of Caution." *Circulation. Heart Failure*, *3* (3), 362–69. doi:10.1161/ CIRCHEARTFAILURE.109.862359.

Cuisset, Thomas. & Thierry, Lefèvre. (2016). "Contemporary Techniques for Catheter-Based Intervention for Hypertrophic Obstructive Cardiomyopathy." *EuroIntervention: Journal of EuroPCR in Collaboration with the Working Group on Interventional Cardiology of the European Society of Cardiology*, *12*, Suppl X (May), X44–47. doi:10.4244/EIJV12SXA9.

Durand, Eric., Elie, Mousseaux., Pierre, Coste., Rémy, Pillière., Olivier, Dubourg., Ludovic, Trinquart., Gilles, Chatellier., Albert, Hagège., Michel, Desnos. & Antoine, Lafont. (2008). "Non-Surgical Septal Myocardial Reduction by Coil Embolization for Hypertrophic Obstructive Cardiomyopathy: Early and 6 Months Follow-Up." *European Heart Journal*, *29* (3), 348–55. doi:10.1093/eurheartj/ ehm 632.

Gersh, Bernard J., Barry, J. Maron., Robert, O. Bonow., Joseph, A. Dearani., Michael, A. Fifer., Mark, S. Link., Srihari, S. Naidu. et al. 2011. "2011 ACCF/AHA Guideline for the Diagnosis and Treatment of Hypertrophic Cardiomyopathy: Executive Summary: A Report of the American College of Cardiology Foundation/American Heart Association Task Force on Practice Guidelines." *Circulation*, *124* (24), 2761–96. doi:10.1161/CIR.0b013e318223e230.

Gimeno, Juan Ramón., María, Teresa Tomé. & William, J. McKenna. (2012). "Alcohol Septal Ablation in Hypertrophic Cardiomyopathy: An Opportunity to Be Taken." *Revista Espanola De Cardiologia (English Ed.)*, *65* (4), 314–18. doi:10.1016/j.recesp.2011.11.021.

Goodwin, J. F., Hollman, A., Cleland, W. P. & Teare, D. (1960). "Obstructive Cardiomyopathy Simulating Aortic Stenosis." *British Heart Journal*, *22* (June), 403–14.

Khouzam, Rami N. & Srihari, S. Naidu. (2014). "Current Status and Future Perspectives on Alcohol Septal Ablation for Hypertrophic Obstructive Cardiomyopathy." *Current Cardiology Reports*, *16* (5), 478. doi:10. 1007/s11886-014-0478-3.

Lafont, A., Durand, E., Brasselet, C., Mousseaux, E., Hagege, A. & Desnos, M. (2005). "Percutaneous Transluminal Septal Coil Embolisation as an Alternative to Alcohol Septal Ablation for Hypertrophic Obstructive Cardiomyopathy." *Heart (British Cardiac Society)*, *91* (1), 92. doi:10.1136/hrt.2004.040790.

Lakkis, N. M., Nagueh, S. F., Dunn, J. K., Killip, D. & Spencer, W. H. (2000). "Nonsurgical Septal Reduction Therapy for Hypertrophic Obstructive Cardiomyopathy: One-Year Follow-Up." *Journal of the American College of Cardiology*, *36* (3), 852–55.

Lawrenz, T. & Kuhn, H. (2004). "Endocardial Radiofrequency Ablation of Septal Hypertrophy. A New Catheter-Based Modality of Gradient Reduction in Hypertrophic Obstructive Cardiomyopathy." *Zeitschrift Fur Kardiologie*, *93* (6), 493–99. doi:10.1007/s00392-004-0097-x.

Lawrenz, Thorsten., Bianca, Borchert., Christian, Leuner., Markus, Bartelsmeier., Jens, Reinhardt., Claudia, Strunk-Mueller., Dorothee, Meyer Zu Vilsendorf., et al. (2011). "Endocardial Radiofrequency Ablation for Hypertrophic Obstructive Cardiomyopathy: Acute Results and 6 Months' Follow-up in 19 Patients." *Journal of the American College of Cardiology*, *57* (5), 572–76. doi:10.1016/j.jacc.2010.07.055.

Liebregts, Max., Pieter, A. Vriesendorp., Bakhtawar, K. Mahmoodi., Arend, F. L. Schinkel., Michelle, Michels. & Jurriën, M. ten Berg. (2015). "A Systematic Review and Meta-Analysis of Long-Term Outcomes After Septal Reduction Therapy in Patients With Hypertrophic Cardiomyopathy." *JACC. Heart Failure*, *3* (11), 896–905. doi:10.1016/j.jchf.2015.06.011.

Liebregts, Max., Pieter, A. Vriesendorp. & Jurrien, M. Ten Berg. (2017). "Alcohol Septal Ablation for Obstructive Hypertrophic Cardiomyopathy: A Word of Endorsement." *Journal of the American College of Cardiology*, *70* (4), 481–88. doi:10.1016/j.jacc.2017.02.080.

Llamas-Esperón, Guillermo A. & Santiago, Sandoval-Navarrete. (2007). "Percutaneous Septal Ablation with Absorbable Gelatin Sponge in Hypertrophic Obstructive Cardiomyopathy." *Catheterization and Cardiovascular Interventions: Official Journal of the Society for Cardiac Angiography & Interventions*, *69* (2), 231–35. doi:10.1002/ccd.20935.

Maron, Barry J. (2007). "Controversies in Cardiovascular Medicine. Surgical Myectomy Remains the Primary Treatment Option for Severely Symptomatic Patients with Obstructive Hypertrophic Cardiomyopathy." *Circulation*, *116* (2), 196–206, discussion 206. doi:10.1161/CIRCULATIONAHA.107.691378.

Maron, Barry J., Julius, M. Gardin., John, M. Flack., Samuel, S. Gidding., Tom, T. Kurosaki. & Diane, E. Bild. (1995). "Prevalence of Hypertrophic Cardiomyopathy in a General Population of Young Adults: Echocardiographic Analysis of 4111 Subjects in the CARDIA Study." *Circulation*, *92* (4), 785–89. doi:10.1161/01.CIR.92.4.785.

Maron, Martin S., Iacopo, Olivotto., Andrey, G. Zenovich., Mark, S. Link., Natesa, G. Pandian., Jeffery, T. Kuvin., Stefano, Nistri., Franco, Cecchi., James, E. Udelson. & Barry, J. Maron. (2006). "Hypertrophic Cardiomyopathy Is Predominantly a Disease of Left Ventricular Outflow Tract Obstruction." *Circulation*, *114* (21), 2232–39. doi:10.1161/CIRCULATIONAHA.106.644682.

Matos, Gabor F., Rasheed, Hammadeh., Christopher, Francois., Richard, McCarthy. & Ferdinand, Leya. (2005). "Controlled Myocardial Infarction Induced by Intracoronary Injection of N-Butyl Cyanoacrylatein Dogs: A Feasibility Study." *Catheterization and Cardiovascular Interventions: Official Journal of the Society for Cardiac Angiography & Interventions*, *66* (2), 244–53. doi:10.1002/ccd.20486.

McCully, R. B., Nishimura, R. A., Tajik, A. J., Schaff, H. V. & Danielson, G. K. (1996). "Extent of Clinical Improvement after Surgical Treatment of Hypertrophic Obstructive Cardiomyopathy." *Circulation*, *94* (3), 467–71.

Morrow, A. G., Reitz, B. A., Epstein, S. E., Henry, W. L., Conkle, D. M., Itscoitz, S. B. & Redwood, D. R. (1975). "Operative Treatment in Hypertrophic Subaortic Stenosis. Techniques, and the Results of Pre and Postoperative Assessments in 83 Patients." *Circulation*, *52* (1), 88–102.

Okutucu, Sercan., Kudret, Aytemir. & Ali, Oto. (2016). "Glue Septal Ablation: A Promising Alternative to Alcohol Septal Ablation." *JRSM Cardiovascular Disease*, *5* (December), 2048004016636313. doi:10. 1177/2048004016636313.

Sorajja, Paul., Steve, R. Ommen., David, R. Holmes., Joseph, A. Dearani., Charanjit, S. Rihal., Bernard, J. Gersh., Ryan, J. Lennon. & Rick, A. Nishimura. (2012). "Survival after Alcohol Septal Ablation for Obstructive Hypertrophic Cardiomyopathy." *Circulation*, *126* (20), 2374–80. doi:10.1161/CIRCULATIONAHA.111.076257.

Steggerda, Robbert C., Kevin, Damman., Jippe, C. Balt., Max, Liebregts., Jurriën, M. ten Berg. & Maarten, P. van den Berg. (2014). "Periprocedural Complications and Long-Term Outcome after Alcohol Septal Ablation versus Surgical Myectomy in Hypertrophic Obstructive Cardiomyopathy: A Single-Center Experience." *JACC. Cardiovascular Interventions*, *7* (11), 1227–34. doi:10.1016/ j.jcin. 2014.05.023.

Vriesendorp, Pieter A., Max, Liebregts., Robbert, C. Steggerda., Arend, F. L., Schinkel, Rik Willems., Folkert, J. Ten Cate., Johan, van Cleemput., Jurriën, M. Ten Berg. & Michelle, Michels. (2014). "Long-Term Outcomes after Medical and Invasive Treatment in Patients with Hypertrophic Cardiomyopathy." *JACC. Heart Failure*, *2* (6), 630–36. doi:10.1016/j.jchf.2014.06.012.

Yoerger, Danita M., Michael, H. Picard., Igor, F. Palacios., Gus, J. Vlahakes., Patricia, A. Lowry. & Michael, A. Fifer. (2006). "Time Course of Pressure Gradient Response after First Alcohol Septal Ablation for Obstructive Hypertrophic Cardiomyopathy." *The American Journal of Cardiology*, *97* (10), 1511–14. doi:10.1016/ j.amjcard.2005.12.040.

In: Hypertrophic Cardiomyopathy
Editor: Ikram Kammoun

ISBN: 978-1-53613-003-4

Chapter 8

HYPERTROPHIC CARDIOMYOPATHY AND PREGNANCY

Emna Bennour*, Ikram Kammoun, Sonia Marrakchi and Salem Kachboura
Department of Cardiology,
Tunis ElManar University, Ariana, Tunisia

ABSTRACT

Pregnancy is considered a potential risk in women with hypertrophic cardiomyopathy (HCM). Most women with hypertrophic cardiomyopathy tolerate pregnancy well. However, women who are symptomatic before pregnancy or who have severe left ventricular outflow tract obstruction or severe systolic left ventricular dysfunction have a higher risk of mortality. Management of pregnant women with HCM is detailed in this chapter.

Keywords: hypertrophic cardiomyopathy, pregnancy, management

---

* Corresponding Author email: bennour_emna@yahoo.fr.

INTRODUCTION

Pregnancy is considered a potential risk in women with hypertrophic cardiomyopathy (HCM). However, its prognosis has not yet been established. The interactions between physiological and hemodynamic changes in pregnancy, such as high cardiac output and HCM pathophysiological changes, including left ventricular outflow obstruction, diastolic dysfunction and myocardial ischemia, may cause high maternal morbidity rates during gestation, delivery and post-partum.

PATHOPHYSIOLOGY OF PREGNANCY

Due to hormonal influences, vasodilation occurs early during pregnancy and causes an increase of maternal blood volume by 40%, pulling an increase from 30 to 50% of the cardiac output.

This increase in cardiac output in the first and second trimester is reached by a larger stroke volume and a rise in heart rate of 10–15 beats per minute. A decrease in systemic vascular resistance in the second trimester causes a diminution in blood pressure (10 mmHg). A rise in certain coagulation factors and a decrease in fibrinolytic activity causes a state of hypercoagulability (Krul et al. 2011).

In pregnant women with HCM, the additional volume load enlarges the ventricular cavity, which theoretically might reduce the LVOT obstruction. However, increased cardiac output tends to counteract this effect and the LVOT gradient increases as gestation advances. The same volume loading increases distension of the left atrium and thereby risk of atrial fibrillation. Volume changes and increased heart rate are not well tolerated by these women, thus aggravating symptoms of dyspnea and may be even leading to left heart failure (Pieper and Walker 2013).

The contracting uterus and rise of catecholamine levels lead to an increase of cardiac output during delivery. There is also an increase in heart rate secondary to blood loss, pain and stress, while the expulsive efforts during delivery tend to diminish venous return. All of these physiological changes lead to an increase in LVOT gradient and shorten the diastolic filling period, therefore increasing the risk of pulmonary edema (Pieper and Walker 2013).

RISK ASSESSMENT

Only a limited number of pregnancies in women with HCM have been described in the literature (Krul et al. 2011).

Most women with HCM tolerate pregnancy well, according to the data available (European Society of Gynecology (ESG) et al. 2011; ICIN working group on Heriditary Heart Diseases 2010). This is explained in most cases by the hypertrophied small left ventricle which can accommodate the physiological increase in blood volume without undue rise in filling pressure.

However, certain patients may have complications (Krul et al. 2011) and a few reported cases of maternal death have occurred, mostly in women who were known to be at very high risk (Pieper and Walker 2013).

A pre-conceptual review is highly recommended in order to identify patients at increased risk (ICIN working group on Heriditary Heart Diseases 2010; Pieper 2011; Gersh et al. 2011). ESC guidelines on managing cardiovascular disease during pregnancy advise that a risk assessment be performed using the modified World Health Organization (WHO) classification (European Society of Gynecology (ESG) et al. 2011).

Most HCM patients are WHO Class II (low risk) or III (increased risk) (Table 1).

Pregnancy is CONTRAINDICATED for a minority of women who present severe systolic LV dysfunction, or severe symptomatic LVOTO (WHO IV), but pregnancy may be possible after relief of LVOTO (Authors/Task Force members et al. 2014). Tomasov reported one of the first cases of a symptomatic patient with severe HCM phenotype and LVOTO, who was first treated with alcohol septal ablation and then had an uncomplicated pregnancy (Tomasov et al. 2017).

Table 1. Modified WHO classification of maternal cardiovascular risk: principles and application (Authors/Task Force members et al. 2014)

Risk class	Risk of pregnancy	Application to HCM
I	No detectable increased risk of maternal mortality and no/mild risk of morbidity	-
II	Small increased risk of maternal mortality or moderate increase in morbidity	Most women with HCM: Mild to moderate LVOTO; asymptomatic with or without medication, well-controlled arrhythmia, normal systolic LV function or mild LV dysfunction
III	Significantly increased risk of maternal mortality or severe morbidity	Severe LVOTO, symptoms or arrhythmias despite optimal medication, moderate systolic LV dysfunction
IV	Extremely high risk of maternal mortality or severe morbidity; PREGNANCY CONTRAINDICATED	Severe systolic LV dysfunction, severe symptomatic LVOTO.

HCM = hypertrophic cardiomyopathy; LV = left ventricle; LVOTO = left ventricular outflow tract obstruction; WHO = World Health Organization.

Echocardiography should be performed on all patients to evaluate ventricular function, mitral regurgitation and LVOTO (Authors/Task Force members et al. 2014).

Exercise testing is an important means of assessing functional capacity, heart rate response and arrhythmias (pre-pregnancy or, in asymptomatic pregnant women, to 80% of predicted maximal heart rate) (European Society of Gynecology (ESG) et al. 2011; Authors/Task Force members et al. 2014).

Medication and follow-up during pregnancy should be discussed and planned with the patient and her partner before conception (European Society of Gynecology (ESG) et al. 2011).

For all women with HCM, genetic counselling is recommended (Authors/Task Force members et al. 2014).

Previous studies in populations of women with both acquired and congenital heart disease have identified several predictors for cardiac complications during pregnancy (Drenthen et al. 2010; Siu et al. 2001). However, these studies cover only a small number of women with HCM. Thus, disease specific series also prove helpful when assessing risk.

In the retrospective study cohort reported by Autore, 100 women known to have HCM with one or more live births (total 199 pregnancies) were included. Two deaths occurred during pregnancy. Both had a particularly high-risk profile and had been strongly advised against becoming pregnant. Maternal mortality is higher in pregnant women with HCM than in the general population. However, absolute maternal mortality is low and appears to be mainly confined to those at particularly high risk (Autore et al. 2002).

Maternal mortality was found to be low too in the few prospective studies available (Siu et al. 2001; Avila et al. 2007).

In a large retrospective study (using questionnaires), Thaman described 271 pregnancies in 127 women with HCM and found that 28.3% reported cardiac symptoms. The majority (90%) of women with symptoms (mainly dyspnea) during pregnancy had already been symptomatic before (Thaman et al. 2003).

In a prospective study by Avila conducted on 35 women with HCM (23 pregnant women and 12 not pregnant), no relationship was found between symptoms before and during pregnancy. In the group of pregnant women, a high percentage of heart failure (30.3%) was observed, particularly during the third trimester, as they presented poor tolerance to pregnancy-related circulatory overload. Hospitalization for treatment of cardiac complications was more frequent in this group, particularly in patients with a family history of HCM (Avila et al. 2007).

In the study conducted by Autore, clinical deterioration occurred more often in women with LVOT obstruction (peak gradient >30 mmHg) than in women without obstruction (25% versus 11%). However, the difference was not statistically significant (Autore et al. 2002). In addition, those who had symptoms prior to pregnancy were more likely to deteriorate than those who did not (42% vs 4%). Other studies also confirmed that deterioration during pregnancy most often occurs in women who are symptomatic before pregnancy (Authors/Task Force members et al. 2014).

In Avila's study there was a small but significant increase in LVOT gradient in pregnancy compared to pre-pregnancy ($p < 0.05$), but no correlation between clinical evolution and the degree of outflow tract obstruction was observed (Avila et al. 2007).

Pregnancy does not appear to aggravate arrhythmias. All patients in the studies by Avila and Thaman who experienced syncope, palpitations or documented arrhythmia had experienced similar symptoms or events before pregnancy. Consequently, arrhythmias before pregnancy are probably predictive of arrhythmias during pregnancy, which is consistent with the literature concerning patients with other heart diseases (Drenthen et al. 2010; Siu et al. 2001; Avila et al. 2007; Thaman et al. 2003). In Avila's series, the occurrence of arrhythmias was similar in a pregnant and a non-pregnant group of women with HCM (Avila et al. 2007).

Schuler reported a retrospective analysis of 19 pregnancies in 14 women with an implantable cardioverter defibrillator (8 women with familial hypertrophic cardiomyopathy). In the group with HCM and an ICD in situ, there were two episodes of paroxysmal arrhythmia (one supraventricular tachycardia and one non-sustained ventricular tachycardia). These tachycardias were detected by the ICD, but no therapy was delivered. One other patient had 2 episodes of sustained ventricular tachycardia which were both terminated by anti-tachycardia pacing (Schuler et al. 2012).

Tanaka reported (Tanaka et al. 2014) on the first study in Japan to investigate cardiovascular events occurring during pregnancy in women with HCM (a total of 27 pregnancies: 23 women with HCM were retrospectively reviewed). The authors indicated that cardiovascular events occurred in 48% of pregnancies, and that arrhythmia (76%) was the most common event. Their new results were that medication before pregnancy and higher CARPREG and ZAHARA scores were risk factors of cardiovascular events during those pregnancies. The CARPREG score is a contemporary assessment of maternal and neonatal risk associated with pregnancy in women with heart disease, and the ZAHARA score is the modified risk score for cardiac complications during completed pregnancies in women with congenital heart disease. The timing of cardiovascular events during pregnancy included in this analysis has not been reported before. The authors proposed that cardiovascular events are most likely to occur either in the first stage of pregnancy, near 30 gestational weeks, or postpartum. Hence, strict control is especially necessary in these 3 peak periods of onset.

Recently, 60 pregnant women with HCM were included into the prospective worldwide Registry of Pregnancy and Cardiac disease (ROPAC) (Goland et al. 2017). The primary endpoint was a major adverse cardiovascular event (MACE): death, heart failure (HF), thrombo-embolic event, and arrhythmia. Baseline and outcome data were analyzed and compared for patients with MACE vs without MACE and for patients with obstructive HCM (41.7% obstructive) vs non-obstructive HCM. No maternal mortality occurred in this cohort. In 14 (23%) patients, at least one MACE occurred. HF was observed in 15% of patients (2 with obstructive and 7 with non-obstructive). Arrhythmia occurred in 12% of patients (6 ventricular tachyarrhythmia and 1 atrial fibrillation). No thrombo-embolic complication occurred. MACE happened most commonly *during the 3rd trimester and postpartum period.* In total, 3 (5.0%) women experienced fetal loss. Women with MACE had a higher rate of emergency caesarean delivery for cardiac reasons (21.4% vs. 0%, P=0.01). No significant differences in pregnancy outcome were found between women with obstructive and non-obstructive HCM. NYHA functional class of ≥ II and signs of HF before pregnancy were associated with the occurrence of MACE.

In conclusion, the few available output data show that, for HCM patients, risk in pregnancy depends highly on pre-pregnancy clinical status. Severe complications are, however, rare. Discussing maternal and fetal risk with the future mother is highly recommended.

Management of Pregnancy and Delivery

As per ESC guidelines, women in WHO Class II should be assessed once every three months by clinical examination and echocardiography.

Women in WHO Class III should be followed monthly or bimonthly in specialized centers by a multidisciplinary team (European Society of Gynecology (ESG) et al. 2011; Authors/Task Force members et al. 2014). Symptomatic status, LV outflow obstruction, arrhythmias and ventricular function must be the main focus of follow-ups. Echocardiography should be performed each trimester or when new symptoms occur.

When medication is prescribed, probable harmful effects to the fetus need to be taken into account. Both doctor and patient should realize that withholding medication from the mother may seriously threaten her health and that of the fetus (e.g., treatment of serious ventricular arrhythmias and anticoagulation therapy for AF). Ultimately, the interests of the mother should prevail (Authors/Task Force members et al. 2014).

B-Blockers should be continued if already used before pregnancy (Authors/Task Force members et al. 2014) (though it is recommended to re-evaluate the need for their use) and side-effects such as growth retardation, neonatal bradycardia or hypoglycemia are usually not severe and can be easily managed.

B-Blockers should be started when new symptoms occur (Krul et al. 2011; European Society of Gynecology (ESG) et al. 2011). Metoprolol is the most widely used; atenolol is not recommended because it has been associated with more growth delay. Whenever B-blockers are prescribed, monitoring fetal growth and the condition of the neonate is recommended.

Diuretics can be prescribed if needed to treat symptoms of dyspnea (Pieper and Walker 2013).

Verapamil and diltiazem are classified by the FDA as class C, meaning that their potential benefits may warrant their use in pregnant women despite potential risks (Authors/Task Force members et al. 2014). Caution is necessary due to the risk of fetal atrioventricular block.

Disopyramide should only be used when potential benefits outweigh risks, since it can cause uterine contractions (Tadmor et al. 1990).

Amiodarone should be used only when absolutely necessary, because of the risk of fetal thyroid toxicity, growth retardation, and neurological adverse effects (European Society of Gynecology (ESG) et al. 2011; Magee et al. 1995; Joglar and Page 1999).

Sotalol can be used during pregnancy (Pieper and Walker 2013).

Poorly tolerated AF can be safely cardioverted during pregnancy. Since a few cases of fetal distress immediately following electrical cardioversion have been described, this procedure should be carried out in facilities where cardiac monitoring and emergency caesarean section are available (Tromp et al. 2011).

Therapeutic anticoagulation with low molecular weight heparin with anti-factor-Xa monitoring (peak anti-Xa level 0.8–1.2U/mL 4–6 hours post-dose) in the first trimester and from the 36th week onwards or VKAs in the second and third trimesteris recommended for paroxysmal or persistent AF (European Society of Gynecology (ESG) et al. 2011). New oral anticoagulants (e.g., dabigatran, rivaroxaban) are not recommended because of proven toxicity in animals and insufficient data in humans (Authors/Task Force members et al. 2014).

When indicated, pacemaker or implantable cardioverter defibrillator (ICD) implantation during pregnancy should be performed with echocardiographic guidance, if possible.

A delivery plan should be discussed by the multidisciplinary team: obstetrician, cardiologist and anesthetist. Planned vaginal delivery is generally preferred although asymptomatic women with mild disease may go into spontaneous labor. Caesarean section is mainly performed for obstetric indications but should be considered in patients with severe LVOTO, pre-term labor while on OAC, or severe heart failure.

Epidural and spinal anesthesia help reduce pain and stress but must be applied judiciously to avoid vasodilation and hypotension, especially when LVOTO is severe. Single-shot spinal anesthesia should be avoided (European Society of Gynecology (ESG) et al. 2011; Authors/Task Force members et al. 2014; Walker et al. 2007).

During delivery, heart rate and rhythm should be monitored in patients with a high risk of developing arrhythmias (Krul et al. 2011). A pulmonary artery Swan-Ganz catheter is best avoided as it increases the risk of thromboembolism and arrhythmias, with little proven benefit. Non-invasive monitoring of cardiac filling and LVOT obstruction can be effectively accomplished by transthoracic echocardiography when required (Ferguson, Paech, and Veltman 2006).

Oxytocin should only be given as a slow infusion in order to avoid hypotension and tachycardia.

Because of the high risk of pulmonary edema due to fluid shifts post-delivery, clinical observation should be continued for 24–48 hours (European Society of Gynecology (ESG) et al. 2011).

There is no need to deactivate an ICD during vaginal delivery (Authors/Task Force members et al. 2014).

The supervision and monitoring of pregnant women with HCM is specified in Table 2.

Table 2. Recommendations for the management of women with hypertrophic cardiomyopathy before and during pregnancy (Pieper and Walker 2013; Authors/Task Force members et al. 2014)

Pre-pregnancy	Clinical symptoms. Echocardiography. Exercise testing. Start medication (beta-blocker, preferably metoprolol) when symptomatic. Risk assessment and counselling. Genetic counselling.
During pregnancy	Follow-up every three months (class II) or monthly/bimonthly (class III). Clinical assessment, echocardiography. Continue beta-blocker or start when symptomatic: monitoring fetal growth and the condition of the neonate is recommended. Prompt treatment of atrial fibrillation: therapeutic anticoagulation with LMWH or vitamin K antagonists depending on the stage of pregnancy is recommended.
Delivery	Vaginal delivery appropriate (it is recommended as the first choice in most patients). Blood pressure and rhythm monitoring. Monitor preload echocardiographically when necessary. Cautious use of epidural or spinal anesthesia. Replace fluid loss, avoid over hydration. Oxytocin only as slow iv infusion. Clinical observation for at least 24h post-delivery.

Conclusion

Pregnancy exposes patients with hypertrophic cardiomyopathy to certain risks, such as arrhythmias and heart failure. Early consultation when contemplating pregnancy is an important aspect of management. Close monitoring by a multidisciplinary team before, during, and in the months after delivery is highly recommended.

References

Authors/Task Force members, Perry M. Elliott, Aris Anastasakis, Michael A. Borger, Martin Borggrefe, Franco Cecchi, Philippe Charron, et al. "2014 ESC Guidelines on Diagnosis and Management of Hypertrophic Cardiomyopathy: The Task Force for the Diagnosis and Management of Hypertrophic Cardiomyopathy of the European Society of Cardiology (ESC)." *European Heart Journal* 35 (39): 2733–79. doi:10.1093/eurheartj/ehu284.

Autore, Camillo, Maria Rosa Conte, Marco Piccininno, Paola Bernabò, Giovanna Bonfiglio, Paolo Bruzzi, and Paolo Spirito. 2002. "Risk Associated with Pregnancy in Hypertrophic Cardiomyopathy." *Journal of the American College of Cardiology* 40 (10): 1864–69.

Avila, Walkiria Samuel, Florence M. Cavalcanti Amaral, Jose Antonio Franchini Ramires, Eduardo Giusti Rossi, Max Grinberg, Maria Rita Lemos Bortolotto, Charles Mady, José Eduardo Krieger, and Marcelo Zugaib. 2007. "Influence of Pregnancy on Clinical Course and Fetal Outcome of Women with Hypertrophic Cardiomyopathy." *Arquivos Brasileiros De Cardiologia* 88 (4): 480–85.

Drenthen, Willem, Eric Boersma, Ali Balci, Philip Moons, Jolien W. Roos-Hesselink, Barbara J. M. Mulder, Hubert W. Vliegen, et al. 2010. "Predictors of Pregnancy Complications in Women with Congenital Heart Disease." *European Heart Journal* 31 (17): 2124–32. doi:10.1093/eurheartj/ehq200.

European Society of Gynecology (ESG), Association for European Paediatric Cardiology (AEPC), German Society for Gender Medicine (DGesGM), Vera Regitz-Zagrosek, Carina Blomstrom Lundqvist, Claudio Borghi, Renata Cifkova, et al. 2011. "ESC Guidelines on the Management of Cardiovascular Diseases during Pregnancy: The Task Force on the Management of Cardiovascular Diseases during Pregnancy of the European Society of Cardiology (ESC)." *European Heart Journal* 32 (24): 3147–97. doi:10.1093/eurheartj/ehr218.

Ferguson, E. A., M. J. Paech, and M. G. Veltman. 2006. "Hypertrophic Cardiomyopathy and Caesarean Section: Intraoperative Use of Transthoracic Echocardiography." *International Journal of Obstetric Anesthesia* 15 (4): 311–16. doi:10.1016/j.ijoa.2005.08.008.

Gersh, Bernard J., Barry J. Maron, Robert O. Bonow, Joseph A. Dearani, Michael A. Fifer, Mark S. Link, Srihari S. Naidu, et al. 2011. "2011 ACCF/AHA Guideline for the Diagnosis and Treatment of Hypertrophic Cardiomyopathy: A Report of the American College of Cardiology Foundation/American Heart Association Task Force on Practice Guidelines." *Circulation* 124 (24): e783-831. doi:10.1161/CIR.0b013e318223e2bd.

Goland, S., I. M. van Hagen, G. Elbaz-Greener, U. Elkayam, A. Shotan, W. M. Merz, S. C. Enar, et al. 2017. "Pregnancy in Women with Hypertrophic Cardiomyopathy: Data from the European Society of Cardiology Initiated Registry of Pregnancy and Cardiac Disease (ROPAC)." *European Heart Journal*. Accessed September 12. doi:10.1093/eurheartj/ehx189.

ICIN working group on Heriditary Heart Diseases. 2010. "Genetic Diagnostics and Genetic Counselling in Hypertrophic Cardiomyopathy (HCM)." *Netherlands Heart Journal: Monthly Journal of the Netherlands Society of Cardiology and the Netherlands Heart Foundation* 18 (3): 144–59.

Joglar, J. A., and R. L. Page. 1999. "Treatment of Cardiac Arrhythmias during Pregnancy: Safety Considerations." *Drug Safety* 20 (1): 85–94.

Krul, Sébastien P. J., Jasper J. van der Smagt, Maarten P. van den Berg, Krystyna M. Sollie, Petronella G. Pieper, and Karin Y. van

Spaendonck-Zwarts. 2011. "Systematic Review of Pregnancy in Women with Inherited Cardiomyopathies." *European Journal of Heart Failure* 13 (6): 584–94. doi:10.1093/eurjhf/hfr040.

Magee, L. A., E. Downar, M. Sermer, B. C. Boulton, L. C. Allen, and G. Koren. 1995. "Pregnancy Outcome after Gestational Exposure to Amiodarone in Canada." *American Journal of Obstetrics and Gynecology* 172 (4 Pt 1): 1307–11.

Pieper, P. G. 2011. "Pre-Pregnancy Risk Assessment and Counselling of the Cardiac Patient." *Netherlands Heart Journal: Monthly Journal of the Netherlands Society of Cardiology and the Netherlands Heart Foundation* 19 (11): 477–81. doi:10.1007/s12471-011-0188-z.

Pieper, P. G., and F. Walker. 2013. "Pregnancy in Women with Hypertrophic Cardiomyopathy." *Netherlands Heart Journal: Monthly Journal of the Netherlands Society of Cardiology and the Netherlands Heart Foundation* 21 (1): 14–18. doi:10.1007/s12471-012-0358-7.

Schuler, Pia K., Anna Herrey, Angie Wade, Ruth Brooks, Donald Peebles, Pier Lambiase, and Fiona Walker. 2012. "Pregnancy Outcome and Management of Women with an Implantable Cardioverter Defibrillator: A Single Centre Experience." *Europace: European Pacing, Arrhythmias, and Cardiac Electrophysiology: Journal of the Working Groups on Cardiac Pacing, Arrhythmias, and Cardiac Cellular Electrophysiology of the European Society of Cardiology* 14 (12): 1740–45. doi:10.1093/europace/eus172.

Siu, S. C., M. Sermer, J. M. Colman, A. N. Alvarez, L. A. Mercier, B. C. Morton, C. M. Kells, et al. 2001. "Prospective Multicenter Study of Pregnancy Outcomes in Women with Heart Disease." *Circulation* 104 (5): 515–21.

Tadmor, O. P., A. Keren, D. Rosenak, M. Gal, M. Shaia, E. Hornstein, H. Yaffe, E. Graff, S. Stern, and Y. Z. Diamant. 1990. "The Effect of Disopyramide on Uterine Contractions during Pregnancy." *American Journal of Obstetrics and Gynecology* 162 (2): 482–86.

Tanaka, Hiroaki, Chizuko Kamiya, Shinji Katsuragi, Kayo Tanaka, Takekazu Miyoshi, Mitsuhiro Tsuritani, Masashi Yoshida, et al. 2014. "Cardiovascular Events in Pregnancy with Hypertrophic

Cardiomyopathy." *Circulation Journal: Official Journal of the Japanese Circulation Society* 78 (10): 2501–6.

Thaman, R., A. Varnava, M. S. Hamid, S. Firoozi, B. Sachdev, M. Condon, J. R. Gimeno, R. Murphy, P. M. Elliott, and W. J. McKenna. 2003. "Pregnancy Related Complications in Women with Hypertrophic Cardiomyopathy." *Heart (British Cardiac Society)* 89 (7): 752–56.

Tomasov, Pavol, Roman Chmel, Marta Novackova, and Josef Veselka. 2017. "Uncomplicated Pregnancy in a Patient Treated With Alcohol Septal Ablation for Hypertrophic Obstructive Cardiomyopathy." *The Canadian Journal of Cardiology* 33 (4): 555.e1-555.e3. doi:10.1016/j.cjca.2016.10.011.

Tromp, C. H. N., A. C. M. Nanne, P. J. M. Pernet, R. Tukkie, and A. C. Bolte. 2011. "Electrical Cardioversion during Pregnancy: Safe or Not?" *Netherlands Heart Journal: Monthly Journal of the Netherlands Society of Cardiology and the Netherlands Heart Foundation* 19 (3): 134–36. doi:10.1007/s12471-011-0077-5.

Walker, D., N. Kaur, R. Bell, and F. Walker. 2007. "Hyperthrophic Obstructive Cardiomyopathy and Pregnancy: University College London Hospital Experience." *Minerva Anestesiologica* 73 (9): 485–86.

INDEX

D

E

F

G

H

I

J

L

M

N

O

P

Q

R

S

T

U

V

W

Y

Z

α